IMMUNOLOGY OF THE EYE
WORKSHOP I:
IMMUNOGENETICS AND
TRANSPLANTATION IMMUNITY

(A Special Supplement to Immunology Abstracts)

The correct manner in which to refer to a paper from
this publication is as follows:

Author of paper, Title of paper
Proceeding 'Immunology of the eye; Workshop: I'
Eds. Steinberg,G.M., Gery,I. and Nussenblatt,R.B.
Sp. Supp. Immunology Abstracts, 1980.
pp ————, 1980

IMMUNOLOGY OF THE EYE
WORKSHOP I:
IMMUNOGENETICS AND
TRANSPLANTATION IMMUNITY

(A Special Supplement to Immunology Abstracts)

Proceedings of a Workshop on Immunogenetics and
Transplantation Immunity (1979 : Chantilly, Va)
December 5-7, 1979
Chantilly, Virginia.

Edited by
George M. Steinberg
Igal Gery
Robert B. Nussenblatt

Sponsored by
National Eye Institute
National Institutes of Health

Information Retrieval Inc.
Washington D.C. and London.

International Standard Book Number 0-904147-25-8
Library of Congress Catalog Card Number 80-83572

Published as a special supplement to:
Immunology Abstracts
Published monthly by Information Retrieval Limited, London.

Published by Information Retrieval Inc.
1911 Jefferson Davis Highway, Arlington, Virginia 22202.

Printed in the United States of America

Contents

Contents (continued)

Contents (continued)

Workshop Planning Committee

Sheldon Cohen, M.D.
Director, Allergic and Immunologic Diseases Program
National Institute of Allergy and Infectious Diseases
National Institutes of Health
Bethesda, MD 20205

Igal Gery, Ph.D.
Visiting Scientist
National Eye Institute
National Institutes of Health
Bethesda, MD 20205

Robert A. Goldstein, M.D., Ph.D.
Chief, Allergic and Clinical Immunology Branch
Immune, Allergic and Immunologic Diseases Program
National Institute of Allergy and Infectious Diseases
National Institutes of Health
Bethesda, MD 20205

Ralph Helmsen, Ph.D.
Acting Chief, Anterior Segment Diseases Branch
National Eye Institute
National Institutes of Health
Bethesda, MD 20205

Thomas O'Brien, Ph.D.
Chief, Anterior Segment Diseases Branch
National Eye Institute
National Institutes of Health
Bethesda, MD 20205

George M. Steinberg, Ph.D.
Director, Cataract Program
Anterior Segment Diseases Branch
National Eye Institute
National Institutes of Health
Bethesda, MD 20205

Editors

Drs. George M. Steinberg, Igal Gery and Robert Nussenblatt with editorial
assistance from: Drs. John Chandler, Sheldon Cohen, Frank Fitch, Bryan
Gebhardt, David Marsh and Arthur Silverstein

List of participants

Dr. Fritz Bach
Immunology Research Center
Box 724
Mayo Memorial Bldg.
University of Minnesota
Minneapolis, MN 55455
612/376-8084

Dr. David BenEzra
Department of Ophthalmology
Hadassah University
Jerusalem, Israel

Dr. G. M. Bleeker
The Netherlands Ophthalmic Institute
Wilhelmina Gastuis
Eerste Helmerstraat 104
Amsterdam 1013
The Netherlands
020-578-3039

Dr. H.I. Cantor
Sidney Farber Cancer Insitute
44 Binney Street, Room 740
Boston, MA 02115
617/732-3348

Dr. Devron H. Char
University of California
3rd and Parnassus Avenue
Room 315
San Francisco, CA 94143
415/666-4096

Dr. John W. Chandler
Eklund Hall
Swedish Hospital Medical
  Center
1102 Columbia
Seattle, WA 98104
206/292-2516

Dr. Carl Cohen
Center for Genetics
University of Illinois
1853 W. Polk Street
Chicago, IL 60612
312/996-2206

Dr. Sheldon G. Cohen
National Institutes of Health
Building 31, Room 7A52
9000 Rockville Pike
Bethesda, MD 20205
301/496-1884

Dr. Donald J. Doughman
Department of Ophthalmology
University of Minnesota
Minneapolis, MN 55455
612/373-8425

Dr. F. Fitch
University of Chicago
Department of Pathology
Chicago, IL 60637
312/947-5451

Dr. Bryan Gebhardt
Department of Ophthalmology
Louisiana State University
Medical Center
New Orleans, LA 70112
504/568-6700

Dr. R. K. Gershon
University School of Medicine
Yale University
310 Cedar Street
New Haven, CT 06510
203/436-2387

Dr. Igal Gery
National Institutes of Health
Building 6, Room 232
9000 Rockville Pike
Bethesda, MD 20205
301/496-4159

Dr. Denis J. Gospodarowicz
University of California
1282 Moffitt Hospital
Cancerr Research Institute
San Francisco, CA 94143
415/666-2165

Dr. Ira Green
National Institutes of Health
Building 10, Room 11N314
9000 Rockville Pike
Bethesda, MD 20205
301/496-6469

Dr. James B. Grogan
University of Mississippi
Medical Center
2500 North State Street
Jackson, MS 39216
601/968-5527

Dr. R. Hong
University of Wisconsin Hospitals
Center for Health Sciences
University of Wisconsin
1300 University Avenue
Madison, WI 53706
608/263-6201, 6200

Dr. Henry J. Kaplan
Emory University Clinic
Section of Ophthalmology
1365 Clifton Rd., N.E.
Atlanta, GA 30322
404/321-0111 ext. 425

Dr. Carolyn Kalsow
University of Louisville
Department of Ophthalmology
Louisville, KY 40202
502/588-5459

Dr. Gordon Klintworth
Department of Pathology
Duke University
Durham, NC 27710
919/684-5116

Dr. D. Marsh
Johns Hopkins Good
Samariton Hospital
5601 Loch Raven Boulevard
Baltimore, MD 21239
301/323-2200 ext 411

Dr. James McCulley
Division of Ophthalmology
Stanford Medical Center
Room a 227
Stanford, CA 94305
415/497-5517

Dr. Linn Murphree
Childrens Hospital of L.A.
4650 Sunset Blvd.
Los Angeles, CA 90054
213/660-2450 ext, 2778

Dr. Robert Nussenblatt
National Institutes
of Health
Building 10, Room 10D09
9000 Rockville Pike
Bethesda, MD 20205
301/496-1243

Dr. Maria Salinas-Carmonia
National Institutes of Health
Bldg. 10, Room 10D09
9000 Rockville Pike
Bethesda, MD 20205
301/496-1243

Dr. E. Shevach
National Institutes
of Health
Building 10, Room 11N315
9000 Rockville Pike
Bethesda, MD 20205
301/496-6449

Dr. Arthur M. Silverstein
Johns Hopkins Hospital
601 North Broadway
Baltimore, MD 21205
301/955-3524

Dr. Richard Simmons
Box 185
Mayo Memorial Building
University of Minnesota
Minneapolis, MN 55455
612/373-8196

Dr. Regina Skelly
National Institutes of Health
Bldg. 6, Room 232
9000 Rockville Pike
Bethesda, MD 20205
301/496-4159

Dr. Walter J. Stark
Johns Hopkins Hospital
Department of Ophthalmology
The Wilmer Institute
601 North Broadway
Baltimore, MD 21205
301/955-5490

Dr. Warren Strober
National Institutes of Health
Bldg. 10, Room 4N114
9000 Rockville Pike
Bethesda, MD 20205
301/496-5387

Dr. Osias Stutman
Sloan Kettering Institute for
  Cancer Research
410 E. 68th Street
New York, NY 10021
212/794-7475

Dr. Hans Wigzell
Department of Immunology
Box 582
BMC
75123 Uppsula, Sweden
018/152000

Dr. Henry J. Winn
Massachusetts General Hospital
Department of Surgery
Boston, MA 02114
617/726-3708

Dr. George M. Steinberg
National Institutes of Health
National Eye Institute
Bldg. 31, Rm 6A52
Bethesda, MD 20205
301/496-5301

Dr. Anita A. Suran
National Institutes of Health
Bldg. 31, Rm 6A52
Bethesda, MD 20205
301/496-5301

Dr. Ralph J. Helmsen
National Institutes of Health
National Eye Institute
Bldg. 31, Rm 6A52
Bethesda, MD 20205
301/496-5984

Preface

Carl Kupfer, M.D.

Director, National Eye Institute, National Institutes of Health, Bethesda, Maryland 20205

The concept for the need of a series of immunology workshops as presently planned by the National Eye Institute (NEI) grew out of several program planning reports which were developed by the National Advisory Eye Council (NAEC). In these documents, the need was clearly identified for an expansion in research effort involving immunological aspects of ocular diseases and for the application of newer concepts and methodology in immunology to the study of the visual system. To accomplish these objectives, the NAEC felt it essential that immunologists active in research outside of the vision field be encouraged to direct their efforts towards research on ocular tissues and ocular systems. An initial approach to the stimulation of dialogue and of collaborative research efforts between vision researchers and immunologists took the form of a grant announcement published by the NEI in the NIH Guide for Grants and Contracts on August 4, 1978, titled "Immunological Aspects of Ocular Disease." A second approach included the development of this workshop series as a joint effort between the National Eye Institute and the National Institute for Allergy and Infectious Diseases (NIAID). In planning sessions between the two Institutes, major research areas were defined which were believed would have the greatest impact upon vision research in the future. Expert investigators who represent each of the subsections of these research areas were identified by NIAID staff members, Drs. Sheldon Cohen and Robert Goldstein, and the

NEI would like to express its appreciation to them for carrying out this important role.

This workshop represents the first in a series of three ocular immunology workshops conducted by the NEI. All workshop participants were divided into task groups to develop a list of research recommendations and priorities perceived by each group as providing the most impetus to vision research.

A second immunology meeting dealing with "Autoimmune Phenomena and Ocular Disorders" was held on March 5-7, 1980, and the third workshop, "Infection, Inflammation and Allergy" was held June 25-27, 1980. The proceedings of these workshops will also be published as special supplements to Immunology Abstracts.

SESSION I

Genetic control of immune response

Summary of Discussion

Included in this section are informal presentations by E. Shevach on the capacity of the immune system to mount a specific immune response[*] and by H. Cantor on the analysis of lymphocyte types involved in the immune reaction, with emphasis on response to tumors.

Specific Immune Response

Immune response (Ir) genes responsible for control have been shown to be thymus dependent. Characteristics of nonresponder animals include failure to demonstrate antibody production and delayed hypersensitivity <u>in vivo</u> and the lack of their cells to proliferate or secrete lymphokine products in <u>in vitro</u> procedures. Ir gene control is effected at the level of interaction of antigen specific T lymphocytes with macrophages or other antigen presenting cells. Thus, activation of a T cell proliferative response of primed T lymphocytes from responder X nonresponder F_1 guinea pigs can only be induced by the antigen-pulsed macrophages from the responder parent but not those taken from a nonresponder parent. When F_1 macrophages are utilized as a source of antigen presenting cells, the proliferative response of F_1 T lymphocytes can be inhibited only by anti-Ia antibody specific for responder antigens but not those of the nonresponder parent, suggesting that the Ir gene product is the Ia antigen. Ir gene control may also be exerted during the interaction of carrier primed T helper cells and

[*] For background literature, see reference 1

hapten primed B lymphocytes in the induction of antibody response. This phenomenon is seen in the primed responder X nonresponder F_1 T helper cells collaborating only with B cells of the responder parent; the defect is identified at the level of the B lymphocyte. While the molecular basis for genetic unresponsiveness in these systems is still unknown, the favored view is that expression of the defect is in both the antigen presenting macrophage and in the B lymphocyte, reflecting a failure of association of the nominal antigen with the Ia antigen gene product. Emphasis was placed upon the role of macrophages in determining the level of immune responsiveness to various antigens. While it is felt that suppressor cells also may be involved in determining levels of immune responsiveness, in most systems studied an exact role has not yet been defined.

Lymphocyte Types

Virtually all natural killer (NK) cells have been shown to carry the Ly5 marker, as exemplified in the nude mouse model where all NK activity is alleviated by treatment with anti Ly5 plus complement. It has been possible to characterize other properties of NK cells by the successful development of a cell clone carrying Ly5 as the Qa2 antigens (Cantor). Good killing capacity is exhibited by these cells in the ratio of one NK:10 target cells. When tested against a battery of lymphoma cells, cloned NK cells have been found to be cytotoxic almost exclusively to virus infected cells. The suggestion that the target components for the NK cells are virus associated is further supported by the finding that killing activity can be specifically inhibited by certain viruses. NK cells also have the capacity to lyse activated B lymphocytes (e.g., LP5-stimulated) but do not affect activated T cells; B cell killing may also be inhibited by lymphoma cells. The existence of cross reacting components on tumor cells and normal spleen cell inhibition of killing by NK cells of E1-4 cells but not YAC cells.

Other work mentioned was that of another group (Bloom) who originally had demonstrated that the capacity of such cell lines as HeLa to kill nude mice was reduced when infected with measles or other viruses. Additionally, when HeLa become infected with viruses in vitro susceptibility to killing by NK cells ensues. The role of interferon (IF) promoting NK cell activity has also been demonstrated in the following approaches: (1) antibodies to IF enhance the growth of tumor cells in nude mice, (2) IF increases the activity of NK cells, and (3) IF can convert cells to Ly5[+] with full killing capacity. Preliminary data further suggest that Ly5[+] cells may release IF which in turn contribute to the recruitment of new NK cells.

A system used to analyze the phenotypes of lymphocytes involved in immunity against cancer was described[2] (Cantor). Derived data indicate that the Ly 1,2,3[+] population contained precursors for cytolytic T cells which become active following conversion to the Ly 2,3[+] phenotype. Ly 1[+] also were found to be active against certain tumors, e.g., MSV-induced sarcoma, probably through secretion of specific antivirion substances. However, Ly 1[+] cells were not active against such tumors as the MLV[+] lymphoma which was affected only by cytolytic Ly 2,3[+] cells.

In consideration of this material it was emphasized that insights concerning the general mechanisms involved in immune responses to antigens such as those relevant to sheep RBC should be applied in studies extended to analyses of immune responses against viruses, bacteria and auto-antigens.

Inquiry was made into whether deficiency in NK activity in humans may be associated with disease and autoimmune phenomena related to increase in NK activity. In this connection it was noted that in the Chediak Higachi syndrome there is a demonstrable lack of NK activity which is also seen in the Beige mouse, an experimental model for this disease. Additionally noted was the increased interferon activity inducing NK activity and the demonstration of increase in interferon levels seen in newborn mice devel-

oping autoimmune diseases. From the clinical standpoint, decreased NK
activity has been associated with HLA 7 and 3 and in patients with primary
biliary cirrhosis. Regarding the Beige mouse, attention was directed to
the report of the high incidence of spontaneous tumors in this model.

Discussion then centered about the relationships between Ly subsets in
mice and subset determinants in humans. Two human T cell subsets have been
described, $(T3+T4)^+$ and $(T3+T5)^+$. The gene product recognized by the
monoclonal antibody T 3 is found on all peripheral cells that are E rosette
positive; it is capable of mediating all T cell functions in vitro including
mitogen reactions. T 3 antibodies block antigen-induced lymphocyte proliferation. The antigen recognized by T 4 antibodies is found on 30
percent of T cells, specifically those that induce B cells to secrete
immunoglobulins and induce cytotoxicity in other T cells. T 5 is found on
20-25 percent of T cells which are cytotoxic effector and suppressor cells
and capable of preventing B cells from producing immunoglobulins. Regarding
the immunochemistry of the Ly system, the Ly 1 product is a polypeptide
with a molecular weight of 60,000 and the Ly 2 product a dimer bridged by
disulfide bonds; each chain having a molecular weight of 30,000. By
immunoprecipitation methods utilizing monoclonal antibodies to human T 4
and T 5, similarity was demonstrated between these components and Ly 1 and
Ly 2,3.

Inquiries were then made into the possible relationships between the
human TH 1-TH 2 and the mouse Ly systems. It was suggested that designations
of the new monoclonal antibodies have significant advantage in the human
system over that noted in the mouse in that they permit the enumeration of
lymphocyte subsets in human disease to be correlated with disease activity.
This is exemplified by the autoantibody found in juvenile rheumatoid
arthritis patients (JRA) where the 30-40 percent of T cells reacting with
JRA autoantibody manifest the equivalent of the Ly 1, 2, 3 subset. In

flare-ups of this disease there is an increased titer of JRA antibody and loss of JRA positive circulating cells and a reversal of these findings coincident with improvement in the clinical state.

Regarding the possibility of whether clones of Ly5 bearing lymphocytes can induce interferon production, it was noted that this is an area of limited information requiring more investigation.

In considering whether other cell clones can be propagated by the same growth factor used to culture NK cells, it was noted that the growth factor recovered from supernatants of a mixed lymphocyte reaction can stimulate the growth of other clones such as T helper and suppressor cells. Because of the complexities of the human system, the question as to whether NK deficiency in humans with tumors is specific to the invading neoplasm or whether a generalized incompetence occurs could not be answered. In the case of secondary infection occuring in cancer patients, increased interferon levels and therefore increased NK levels may be induced. However, there is the exception of low NK activity in patients with Hodgkins disease. Belief was expressed that because of the great variability in NK levels such questions may only be answered by a large scale prospective clinical trial relating NK activity to the incidence of neoplasm. Specifically, regarding NK activity in ocular disease, there has been a preliminary report of slight decrease in NK activity associated with retinoblastoma.

In summarizing the essence of these discussions the marked diversity and specificity of the NK system was emphasized and it was further pointed out that virus associated lipoproteins are the most likely target antigens.

REFERENCES

1. Shevach, E.M. 1978. The guinea pig I region. A functional analysis of Ia-Ir associations. Springer Seminars in Immunopathol. 1:207.
2. Leclerc, J.C., and H. Cantor. 1980. T cell-mediated immunity to oncornavirus-induced tumors. I. Ly phenotype of precursor and effector cytolytic T lymphocytes. J. Immunol. 124:846.

SESSION II.

GENETICS OF HISTOCOMPATIBILITY

Moderator: Ethan Shevach

The major histocompatibility complex and T lymphocyte activation

Fritz H.Bach, M.D.

Immunobiology Research Center and Departments of Laboratory Medicine/Pathology and Surgery, University of Minnesota

ABSTRACT

The major histocompatibility complex in mouse and man has been divided into a number of regions based on a marker locus for each of the regions. Major histocompatibility genes code for molecules that express different "types" of determinants based on the response of functionally disparate T lymphocyte subpopulations to those determinants. Discussed in this paper is our present state of knowledge regarding the loci and regions of H-2, the major histocompatibility complex in mouse, and HLA, the major histocompatibility complex in man. Also, the response of helper T lymphocytes and cytotoxic T lymphocytes to MHC encoded antigens.

INTRODUCTION

A wide variety of biological phenomena have been related to genes of the major histocompatibility complex (MHC), including genetic control of the strongest H antigens and the activation of functionally disparate T lympho-cyte subpopulations by those antigens.[1,2] Much of the information that has been gained has used either mouse or man as the experimental species, al-though studies in guinea pig, rat and rhesus monkey have all contributed. It is my purpose in this paper to review the MHC in both mouse and man with respect to detectable markers encoded by genes of the MHC as well as to discuss T lymphocyte reactivity to various antigens of the MHC.

The major approaches used for detection of MHC encoded antigens involves serological methods; there are serologically detected determinants that are recognized on essentially all cells of the body and others that have an apparently more restricted tissue distribution. In addition there are cel-lular methods, involving activation of T lymphocytes, that can be used to define MHC encoded determinants; here, also, determinants can be divided into two categories including those that activate much of the proliferative re-sponse in a primary mixed leukocyte culture (MLC) in which the donors of the responding and stimulating cells for the MLC differ by an entire MHC, and those that are recognized by cytotoxic T lymphocytes.

There is substantial evidence to suggest that determinants recognized

Table 1

Designations for MHC Encoded Antigens

Method	Mouse		Man	
	K/D	I	ABC	D
Serologic	SD	Ia	SD	DR
Cellular Response	CD[*]	LD	CD	LD

[*]See discussion in text on distribution of LD and CD.

serologically and those recognized by T lymphocytes are not identical. Conceptually, thus, we must deal with two methods of detection: serologic and cellular, with two different "types" of antigens recognized by each of the methods. In order to have a uniform nomenclature that allows us to refer to these various types of determinants in any species, the designations given in Table 1 have been used. These differentiate between the serologically defined antigens found ubiquitously, on essentially all cell surfaces, as the S determinant (SD) antigens; and the serologically detected antigens with a much more limited tissue distribution encoded by different genes by the MHC referred to as I-region associated (Ia or Ia-like) in mouse and some other species and D related (DR) in man. The antigens detected by T lymphocyte reactivities are referred to as L determinants (LD) and C determinants (CD) as listed.

H-2 -- THE MAJOR HISTOCOMPATIBILITY COMPLEX IN MOUSE

A schematic representation of the H-2 complex is given in Figure 1. The recombinational frequency between H-2K and H-2D is approximately 0.005. The H-2 complex is divided into a number of different regions, and subregions, each of which has a "marker locus". The exact boundaries of a region in a strain depend on recombinational events defining that region. In those cases where two or more strains exist in which one can designate a given region, the boundaries are quite likely different in the different mouse strains. As such, it is to be anticipated that new loci will be mapped between the presently designated marker loci and new regions thus established.

There are two classically defined H-2 SD loci, H-2K and H-2D, plus a more recently defined locus, H-2L[3], that appear to fit the category of loci the genes of which code for S determinant, or SD, antigens. Relatively little is known about the H-2L locus at this stage and I shall thus discuss

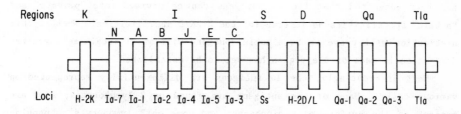

Figure 1. A schematic representation of the H-2 complex including the currently recognized loci. See text for discussion.

H-2K and H-2D. Both of these loci are very highly polymorphic. Associated with each allele of H-2K or H-2D there is what is referred to as a "private" specificity as well as several "public" specificities. These terms refer to the frequency of finding a given specificity in association with the H-2K/D alleles. The private specificities are essentially unique to a given allele of one or the other locus whereas the public specificities can be found in association with several alleles of both H-2K and H-2D.

The I region, initially so designated because of the presence of an immune response (Ir) locus mapping to that segment of the complex[4], has been subdivided into five subregions, A, B, J, E and C. The various regions and subregions of H-2 currently recognized, thus, include the following (with the marker locus for each given in parentheses): K (H-2K), I-A (Ia-1), I-B (Ia-2), I-J (Ia-4), I-E (Ia-5), I-C (Ia-3), S (Ss) and D (H-2D). Listed in Figure 1 is the segment of chromosome immediately to the right of H-2D. Three different loci refered to as Qa-1, Qa-2, and Qa-3[5] have been mapped between H-2D and the Tla locus, which maps one recombinational unit to the right of H-2D. Also shown is a proposed addition to the I region loci (and subregions), I-N, the existence of which Dr. Colleen Hayes and I[6] have recently proposed. The designations for both the subregion and the locus must be considered provisional. I-N is included since possible differences between two strains for I-N could be important in any study of differences in function subserved by K vs. I region encoded antigens.

Although the I region, and in fact the first two subdivisions of that region, were mapped on the basis of Ir genes[4,7], the presently accepted marker loci for each of the I subregions are loci coding for Ia antigens[8-10]. Approximately 50 different antigenic determinants that are listed as Ia have been described; some of these are found associated with only a single sub-region of I whereas others have not been as precisely mapped genetically. It has been suggested that the Ia antigens can be divided into "private" and "public" specificities as is true for the H-2K/D specificities. Whether this distinction will prove to be a useful one and will still obtain as a greater dissection is made of the region has yet to be established.

Most interestingly, the Ia antigens are differentially represented on various cells. Many of the antigens are found on B lymphocytes; some are present on the surface of macrophages; and some on T lymphocyte subpopulations. Cell populations have been subclassified on the basis of their Ia antigen phenotype. Thus, for instance, macrophages are classified as Ia-positive and Ia-negative with presumably different functional abilities ascribed to each of the populations[11]. T lymphocytes have been demonstrated to carry Ia antigens associated with the different subregions of I depending on the functional classification of the T lymphocyte. Although not an absolute association, the Ia antigens of the I-A subregion have in large measure been related to helper T lymphocytes and to a T helper factor whereas the antigens of the I-J subregion have been related to suppressor T lymphocytes[12] and a suppressor factor[13].

Given the differential expression of the Ia antigens associated with the different subregions, the expression of the Ia antigens on one set of cells, such as T lymphocytes and not on another, such as B lymphocytes has been investigated. One line of evidence suggesting such to be the case relates to the I-J encoded Ia antigens which are found on T suppressor cells but not on various other subpopulations of T lymphocytes[12].

Dr. Colleen Hayes and I have investigated this matter further by using the observation that Con A activated thymocytes express Ia antigens[14, 15]. We have used Con A activated thymocytes as the immunogen in a number of different genetic combinations differing by only certain subregions of I. Following the immunization protocol we have tested the resultant sera for their reactivity with T lymphocytes and B lymphocytes. In at least some of these cases, the Ia antigens detected are expressed only on T lymphocytes and not on B lymphocytes (other cell types have not been extensively investigated); further, of the T lymphocytes isolated by different methods, only small subpopulations are reactive with the serum directed at antigens associated with any single subregion of I. This type of approach may be one example of a method of obtaining results that will allow a finer dissection of the I region and understanding of the differential expression of the Ia antigens. The sera produced in this manner have been shown to react with certain functionally active subpopulations[16, 17].

Immune response genes, as already mentioned, map to the I region. It has been suggested that there are Ir loci in the I-A, I-B and I-E/C subregions. (The presumed E and C subregions of I are often written as E/C since it is difficult with present sera to establish the existence of the two separate marker loci for E and C.) In some cases immune responsiveness is the result of complementation between genes mapping in the I-A and I-E/C subregions, for example. The genes mapping in the right portion of the I region are usually referred to as alpha, and those mapping in I-A as beta, genes. In addition to the immune response genes there are genes that control the generation of suppressor cell responses referred to as immune suppression (Is) genes; here, also, complementation has been described[18].

An important consideration for some of the studies in man is the finding that complementing Ir genes are more effective when they are in cis than in trans configuration[19]. This finding can be evoked to explain the linkage disequillibrium found between certain genes of the MHC in man.

The Ss locus codes for the presence of the fourth component of complement[20]. The different alleles of the Ss locus are associated with high or low levels of this component.

The Qa loci[5] are not classically included as a part of the H-2 complex although their inclusion or exclusion to some extent would have to be considered quite arbitrary. The antigens encoded by genes of these loci appear to be differentiation antigens, in the same sense that the Ia antigens are. Anti-Qa-1 sera, for instance, are able to subdivide the proliferating cells in a primary MLC into Qa-1 positive and Qa-1 negative cells[21]. Likewise, this marker has been used to delineate two subpopulations, one of which is active in the feedback suppression phenomenon, the other which is not[22].

The exact relationship of the molecules carrying the Ia determinants to the genetic control of immune response by I region genes is not established. Various models have been put forth that would involve these "Ia molecules" in terms of antigen presentation, cell interactions involving the Ia carrying molecules as both the factors functioning for help or suppression and as the receptors for these factors, and others.

HLA--THE MAJOR HISTOCOMPATIBILITY COMPLEX IN MAN

Presented in Figure 2 is a schematic representation of the HLA complex. In man, as in mouse, serologic and cellular methods have been used for the definition of the various antigens and molecules encoded by HLA genes. The HLA A, B, and C loci code for antigens that are present on essentially all

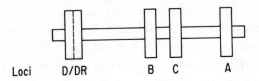

Figure 2. A schematic representation of the HLA complex. See text for discussion.

cells of the body that show sequence homology with the H-2K/D antigens. The HLA-D locus was first defined using cellular techniques, i.e. proliferation in a primary MLC; thus, the antigens associated with HLA-D that can be detected by serological methods have been referred to as the DR (D related) antigens. The DR antigens are thought to be homologues of the Ia antigens.

Presented in Table 2 are the presently recognized antigens of HLA both as detected by serologic methods and by the primary mixed leukocyte culture response to homozygous typing cells. As noted, the HLA-A and -B loci are very markedly polymorphic with a continuing finer definition of determinants that can be recognized by different sera. The HLA-C locus does not appear to be as polymorphic as HLA-A and -B.

The HLA-D locus is formally defined by response in a primary mixed leukocyte culture to homozygous typing cells (HTCs). The HTC technique involves the use of stimulating cells that are homozygous for HLA-D antigen(s). The rationale behind HTC testing that if a given individual does not carry the antigen(s) present on the HTC, then there should be a strong response by the cells of that individual to that particular HTC. If, on the other hand, a different individual carries the antigen(s) present on that HTC, then there should be a relatively weak, or absent, response by the cells of that individual to the same HTC.

Although the results obtained with most HTCs, that are either genotypically or simply phenotypically homozygous for HLA-D, are not as "clean" as suggested by the prototype results suggested above, it is possible to obtain useful information and a number of different HLA-D antigens (or antigenic clusters) have been defined utilizing HTCs. These are listed as HLA-DW1 through DW11 in Table 2.

Seven different antigens have been recognized serologically that are associated with the HLA-D locus and are referred to as HLA-DRW1 through

Table 2

HLA Encloded Antigens

D		B		C	A	
W1	RW1	W4		W1	1	W19
W2	RW2	W6		W2	2	W23
W3	RW3			W3	3	W24
W4	RW4	5	W35	W4	9	W30
W5	RW5	7	W38	W5	10	W31
W6	RW6	8	W39	W6	11	W32
W7	RW7	12	W41		25	W33
W8		13	W42		26	W34
W9		14	W44		28	W36
W10		15	W45		29	W43
W11		17	W46			
		18	W47			
		27	W48			
		37	W49			
		40	W50			
		W16	W51			
		W21	W52			
		W22	W53			
			W54			

HLA-DRW7. Very recently, a second series of HLA-DR antigens has been proposed to exist that would appear to be distinct from the series involving
HLA-DRW1 through DRW7. The evidence for the existence of this second series
will be further analyzed at the 8th International Histocompatibility Workshop
in 1980.

The relationship of the HLA-D to the HLA-DR antigens is not well eluci-
dated. Whereas a given HLA-D antigen is most frequently found in a given
population with a given HLA-DR antigen (for the sake of convenience, one
refers, in most instances, to an individual having HLA-DW1 as also having
HLA-DRW1), there is evidence to suggest that the determinants recognized by
cellular response and serologically are different. This evidence is based
both on a very few putative recombinants within HLA-D[23, 24] region as well as
the existence within Caucasians, and other populations of associations between HLA-DR and HLA-D other than those most commonly found in the Caucausian

population. Thus, for instance, in the Oriental population, the antigen HLA-DRW2 is frequently found with the D specificity referred to as DHO. Whereas this association is also found in the Caucasian population, the most common association in Caucasians with DRW2 is, by convention, the DW2 specificity.

An additional method that has provided information about the HLA-D region has been primed LD typing (PLT)[25, 26]. This method uses "sensitization" of lymphocytes in vitro in a primary mixed leukocyte culture in which donor of responding and stimulating cells differ by only a single HLA haplotype. The cells resulting 10 days following the initiation of the primary MLC are thought to represent "secondary-type" responding cells that will give a response, measured by 24 or 48 hours, to those antigens initially recognized by the responding cells on the stimulating cells during the sensitization phase. Although PLT reagents can respond to antigens other than those encoded by the HLA-D region, most of the responses are associated with HLA-D region encoded determinants.

PLT reagents can be prepared, each against a different HLA-D haplotype, and used to "define" PL antigens associated with HLA-D. A number of different PL antigens have been defined in this manner, most of which are highly associated with a given HLA-D antigenic cluster.

The PLT test can be used to detect both antigens associated with HLA-D and those associated with HLA-DR. This can be demonstrated by studying the situation mentioned immediately above in which DRW2 is associated with DHO in Orientals but primarily with DW2 in caucasions. PLT reagents can be prepared against either the DRW2-DW2 or the DRW2-DHO complex and then tested for their responsiveness to each of these two types of stimulating cells. Under these conditions, there appears to be a clear response associated with DRW2, however the magnitude of the response is also affected by the presence of the priming D specificity on the restimulating cells. Further information regarding reactivity with D, or a factor associated with D, is obtained if priming is done against only DW2 or DHO, with respect to these determinants. Under these conditions the resulting PLT reagents react only with DW2 and not with DHO if primed to DW2 and vice versa[27] (see Table 3).

A finer analysis of D associated antigens is promised by the recent advent of cloning of PLT cells. Day 4 blasts were isolated from a regular PLT reagent during the sensitization phase and then cloned in the presence of T cell growth factor (TCGF). Under these conditions, presumed single precursor cells can be grown to very large numbers. In many cases the resulting

Table 3

PLT Response to HLA-D and -DR

Sensitization MLC[+]		Restimulation with:	
Responder	Stimulator	DRW2/DW2	DRW2/DHO
DRWX/DWX[*]	DRW2/DW2	++++	+++
DRWX/DWX	DRW2/DHO	+++	++++
DRW2/DHO	DRW2/DW2	+++	±
DRW2/DW2	DRW2/DHO	±	+++

[*] DRWX and DWX refers to any DR or D antigen other than DRW2 and DW2 or DHO

[+] Adapted from Reinsmoen et al. (27). Semi-quantitative results obtained with PLT reagents sensitized either to both DRW2 and DW2 or DRW2 and DHO or presumably "only" to DW2 and DHO when the responding cell donor is DRW2 positive. The slightly greater restimulation response seen following sensitization to both DRW2 and either DW2 and DHO when the restimulating cell carries the sensitizing D antigen as well as DRW2 is difficult to establish with a high degree of confidence. However, the very strong response to either DW2 or DHO when priming was done against the DW2 and DHO respectively (when the responding cell donor was DRW2 positive) is very clear.

"monoclonal" PLT reagents give highly significant PLT-type responses providing a dissection of the D region hitherto unavailable with cellular reagents[28] (Table 4). The use of cloned PLT reagents must be considered at its inception and thus much further analysis is needed to evaluate is practical usefulness.

CELLULAR RESPONSE TO MHC ENCODED ANTIGENS

Much of the interest relating to different "types" of antigens that are encoded by MHC genes is based on the differential response of helper T lymphocytes (T_h) and cytotoxic T lymphocytes (T_c) to antigens associated with different subregions of the MHC.

The findings can be summarized (1) as follows. (1) H-2 I region encoded LD antigens are primarily responsible for activating the vast majority of the proliferating cells in a primary MLC where the donors of the responding and stimulating cells differ by the entire MHC. (2) The strongest cytotoxic responses are aimed at K/D encoded CD antigens although both I region and Qa region encoded CD antigens exist. (3) The combined presence of K and/or D

Table 4

Proliferative response of non-cloned PLT vs. limiting
dilution "cloned" alloactivated cells

$\underline{A}_x$	$\underline{B}_x$	$\underline{C}_x$	$\underline{D}_x$	Restimulating Cells		Responding Cells	
Original PLT				173	5152	831	207
"Clones"							
	40-10E			543	6000	536	375
	40-7E			641	44681	906	489
	40-8E			576	3842	2313	710
	40-4E			814	4634	2475	683
	40-9D			881	999	993	742

"Clones" were obtained from limiting dilution of day 4 MLC blast cells
and were grown in Terasaki microtiter wells in the presence of feeder layers
and TCGF. The cells were derived from wells which received on the average 40
cells per well at the time of dilution into Terasaki plates. 40-9D is an
example of a clone giving no proliferative response.

region differences plus an I region encoded difference on the stimulating
cells results in the generation of a much stronger cytotoxic response than do
K or D region encoded antigens alone. This phenomenon was referred to as
LD-CD collaboration.

In order to evaluate the cellular response counterpart of LD-CD collaboration at the antigenic level requires familiarity with the differentiation
antigens on the various T lymphocyte subpopulations as defined with anti-Ly
sera. There are three types of lymphocytes to be considered: first, Ly 1+2-
(Ly 1) T_h cells, second, Ly 1-2+ (Ly 2) T_c; and third, Ly 1+2+ (Ly 1,2) cells
that will be discussed further below.

The hypothesis that T_h and T_c are differentially responsive to I region
encoded LD antigens and K/D region encoded CD antigens was based on both
genetic studies using monolayer adsorption[29] and use of anti-Ly sera[30-32].
The monolayer adsorption studies permitted a separation of the great majority
of proliferating cells into a non-adherent fraction which was not cytotoxic
and a smaller percentage of the cells that were adherent and included the

cytotoxic cells. Studies with the anti-Ly sera showed that the great majority of the proliferating cells were of the Ly 1 phenotype, and presumably
included T_h, with the cytotoxic cells included in the Ly 2 population. Most
importantly, and paralleling the phenomenon at the antigenic level of LD-CD
collaboration, it was a collaborative event between the Ly 1 T_h and the Ly 2
T_c that led to the generation of the strong cytotoxic response directed at
K/D encoded CD antigen. The cellular model that evolved from these studies
is shown in the lower half of Figure 3.

A fundamental question, for which we have only recently obtained preliminary data[30, 31], concerns the nature of the cellular response to K/D
region encoded allo-antigens without the concomitant presence of the I region
encoded, LD, allo-antigens that are known to activate the Ly 1 T_h. Under
these circumstances, it appears, that an Ly 1,2 cell is essential as a precursor to allow the cytotoxic response to proceed (i.e. a mixture of Ly 1 and
Ly 2 cells, obtained by separate elimination of Ly 2 and Ly 1 cells respectively, will not collaborate to produce an anti-K/D region response. Since a
large percentage of the effector cytotoxic T lymphocytes that are generated
under these genetic conditions are of the Ly 1,2 phenotype it is reasonable
to suggest that the Ly 1,2 precursor functions as a precursor T_c. We have
suggested on this basis that there are alternative pathways of T lymphocyte
activation and that the presence of an I region encoded LD stimulus may

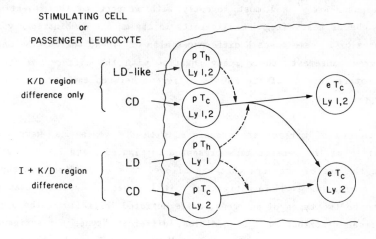

Figure 3. Cellular model for T lymphocyte response to alloantigens.

determine the balance between the two pathways (see Figure 3).

It would thus seem that there are different types of antigens encoded by MHC genes, the LD antigens encoded in the H-2 I region and the CD antigens primarily encoded in the K/D regions. The pathways of T lymphocyte differentiation that are utilized to generate T_c appear to differ depending on the presence of I region encoded differences on the stimulating cells.

MUTANTS OF H-2

The spontaneous mutants of H-2 were first detected by Bailey and co-workers[35]. It is most likely that at least some of the mutants carry K/D molecules that differ from the parental strain by only a single amino acid[36]. These mutants have been of great interest since the mutation frequency is very high and the biological phenomena related to the mutation have been varied and interesting. The mutants are detected based on their ability to reject skin grafts from the parental strain and vice-versa[35]; MLC studies have demonstrated that strong cytotoxic responses are generated in these combinations[37, 38].

Mention of the mutants is included in this paper simply to caution that it appears ill-advised to use the H-2K or D mutants as equivalents to a K or D "region" difference in recombinant strains. In many respects the parent-mutant combinations do not behave as do combinations differing by a K or D region. This is true with regard to the intensity of the in vitro generated cytotoxic response that results in MLC[37, 38], with regard to the ability of mutant vs. K region differences to activate thymocytes to generate a cytotoxic response[39, 40] and most recently with respect to the rejection of thyroid lobe or heart fragment allografts in the mutant combinations vs. H-2 differences or in some cases K differences also[41]. Thus, whereas the mutants are of great interest, their ready equation with the differences included when an entire segment of the MHC is different between two strains does not appear appropriate.

SUMMARY

A variety of markers are associated with MHC genes that have allowed construction of the genetic maps presented in Figures 1 and 2. Primarily it has been the use of antisera that has allowed this dissection. In the process of performing such investigations, it has become apparent that there appear to be two types of antigens, differentiated initially on the basis of their tissue distribution. In addition, different "types" of antigens are differentially active in stimulating Ly 1 T_h and Ly 2 T_c cells.

The focus of this paper has been on a description of these antigens, analyzed both by serological and cellular means, and the functions that the antigens appear to subserve in terms of their activation of T lymphocyte subpopulations. Major areas of investigation relating to immune response, immune suppression, the relationship of MHC encoded markers to disease susceptibility and others have not been included in this review.

ACKNOWLEDGEMENTS

This work was supported by NIH grants AI 08439, CA 09106, CA 16836, and AI 15588. This is paper No. 223 from the Immunobiology Research Center, University of Minnesota, Minneapolis, MN 55455.

REFERENCES
1. Bach, F. H., M. L. Bach, and P. M. Sondel. 1976. Differential function of major histocompatibility complex antigens in T-lymphocyte activation. In: Leukocyte Membrane Determinants Regulating Immune Reactivity, Acad. Press, N.Y., p. 417.
2. Klein, J. 1975. Biology of the Mouse Histocompatibility-2 Complex. Principles of Immunogenetics Applied to a Single System. Springer-Verlag New York, Inc., New York.
3. Morello, D., C. Neuport-Sautes, and P. Demant. 1977. Topographical relationships among H-2 specificities controlled by the D region. Immunogenetics 4: 349.
4. McDevitt, H. O., B. D. Deak, D. C. Shreffler, J. Klein, and J. H. Stimpfling. 1972. Genetic control of the immune response. Mapping of the Ir-1 locus. J. Exp. Med. 135: 1259.
5. Stanton, T. H., and E. A. Boyse. 1976. A new serologically defined locus, Qa-1, in the Tla-region of the mouse. Immunogenetics 3: 525.
6. Hayes, C. E., and Bach, F. H. 1979. I-N: A newly described H-2 locus between K and I-A. J. Exp. Med., in press.
7. Lieberman, R., and W. Humphrey Jr. 1972. H-2 linked immune responses (Ir) genes: Separation of Ir genes for IgG and IgA allotypes in the mouse. Fed. Proc. 31: 777.
8. Shreffler, D. C. and C. S. David. 1975. The H-2 major histocompatibility complex and the I immune response region: Genetic variation, function, and organization. Adv. Immunol. 20: 125.
9. David, C. S. 1976. Serologic and genetic aspects of murine Ia antigens. Transplant. Rev. 30: 299.
10. Cullen, S. E. and B. D. Schwartz. 1976. An improved method for isolation of H-2 and Ia alloantigens with immunoprecipitation induced by protein-A-bearing Staphlococci. J. Immunol. 117: 136.
11. Cowing, C., B. Schwartz, and H. Dickler. 1978. Macrophage Ia antigens I. Macrophage populations differ in their expression of Ia antigen. J. Immunol. 120: 378.
12. Murphy, D. B., L. A. Herzenberg, K. Okumura, L. A. Herzenberg and H. O. McDevitt. 1976. A new I subregion (I-J) marked by a locus (Ia-4) controlling surface determinants on suppressor T lymphocytes. J. Exp. Med. 144: 699.
13. Tada, T., M. Taniguchi, and C. S. David. 1976. Properties of the antigen-specific suppressive T-cell factor in the regulation of antibody synthesis of the mouse IV special subregion. Assignment of the gene(s) that codes for the suppressive T-cell factor in the H-2 histocompatibility complex. J. Exp. Med. 144: 713.
14. Hayes, C. E., and Bach, F. H. 1978. T cell specific murine IA antigens: Serology of I-J and I-E subregion specificities. J. Exp. Med. 148: 692.

15. Hayes, C. E., and Bach, F. H. 1979. T-cell-specific murine Ia antigens. II: Further studies on I-J subregion specificities. J. Immunol., in press.

16. Swienkosz, J.E., Marrack, P., and Kappler, J.W. 1979. Functional analysis of T cells expressing Ia antigens. I. Demonstration of helper T cell heterogeneity. J. Exp. Med., in press.

17. Hayes, C., Macphail, S., and Bach, F. H. 1979. Generation of primary cytotoxic response in vitro to non-MHC antigens. Submitted for publication.

18. Debre, P., C. Waltenbaugh, M. Dorf, B. Benacerraf. 1976. Genetic control of specific immune suppression. III. Mapping of H-2 complex complementing genes controlling immune suppression by the random co-polymer L-Glutamic Acid^{50}-L-Tyrosine^{50} (GT). J. Exp. Med. 144: 272.

19. Dorf, M. E., P. H. Mauer, C. F. Merryman, B. Benacerraf. 1976. Inclusion group systems and cis-trans effects in responses controlled by the two complementing Ir-GLφ genes. J. Exp. Med. 143: 889.

20. Meo, T., Krasteff, T., and Shreffler, D. C. 1975. Immunochemical characterization of murine H-2 controlled Ss (serum substance) protein through identification of its human homologue as the fourth component of complement. Proc. Natl. Acad. Sci. USA 72: 4536.

21. Stanton, T., C. Calkins, J. Jandinski, D. Schendell, O. Stutman, H. Cantor, and E. Boyse. 1978. The Qa-1 antigenic system. Relation of Qa-1 phenotypes to lymphocyte sets, nitrogen responses and immune functions. J. Exp. Med. 148: 963.

22. Cantor, H., J. Hugenberger, L. McVay-Boudreau, D. Eardley, J. Kemp, F. Shen, and R. Gershon. 1978. Immunoregulatory circuits among T cell sets. Identification of a subpopulation of T helper cells that induce feedback inhibition. J. Exp. Med. 148: 871.

23. Reinsmoen, N., H. Noreen, P. Friend, E. Giblett, L. Greenberg and J. Kersey. 1979. Anomalous mixed lymphocyte culture reactivity between HLA-A, B, C, DR identical siblings. Tissue Antigens 13: 19-34.

24. In Histocompatibility Testing 1977. 1978. Munksgaard, Copenhagen, p. 360.

25. Sheehy, M. H., P. M. Sondel, M. L. Bach, R. Wank, and F. H. Bach. 1975. LD (lymphocyte defined) typing: A rapid assay with primed lymphocytes. Science 188: 1308.

26. Bach, F. H., E. K. Jarrett-Toth, C. J. Benike, C. Y. Shih, and E. A. Valentine. 1977. Primed LD typing: Reagent preparation and definition of the HLA-D region antigens. Scand. J. Immunol. 6: 469.

27. Reinsmoen, N. L., H. J. Noreen, T. Sasazuki, M. Segall, and F. H. Bach. 1979. Roles of HLA-DR and HLA-D antigens in haplotype-primed LD typing reagents. 13th International Leucocyte Culture Conference, Ottawa, Canada. Elsevier/North-Holland and Biomedical Press, in press.

28. Bach, F. H., H. Inouye, J. A. Hank, and B. J. Alter. 1979. Human T lymphocyte clones reactive in primed lymphocyte typing and cytotoxicity. Nature 281: 307.

29. Bach, F. H., M. Segall, K. S. Zier, P. M. Sondel, and B. J. Alter. 1973. Cell mediated immunity: Separation of cells involved in recognitive and destructive phases. Science 180: 403.

30. Kisielow, P., J. A. Hirst, H. Shiku, P. C. L. Beverly, and M. K. Hoffman. 1975. Ly antigens as markers for functionally distinct subpopulations of thymus-derived lymphocytes of the mouse. Nature 253: 219.

31. Cantor, H., and E. A. Boyse. 1975. Functional subclasses of T lymphocytes bearing different Ly antigens. I. The generation of functionally distinct T-cell subclasses is a differentiative process independent of antigen. J. Exp. Med. 141: 1376.

32. Cantor, H., and E. A. Boyse. 1975. Functional subclasses of T lymphocytes bearing different Ly antigens. II. Cooperation between subclasses of Ly+ cells in the generation of killer activity. J. Exp. Med. 141: 1390.

33. Bach, F. H., and B. J. Alter. 1978. Alternative pathways of T lymphocyte activation. J. Exp. Med. 148: 829.

34. Alter, B. J., and F. H. Bach. 1979. Speculations on alternative pathways of T lymphocyte response. Scand. J. Immunol. 10: 87.

35. Bailey, D. W., G. D. Snell and M. Cherry. 1971. Complementation and serological analysis of an H-2 mutant. Proc. of the Symp. on Immunogenetics of the H-2 System. Karger AG, Basel Switzerland, p. 155.

36. Brown, H. L., and S. G. Nathenson. 1977. Structural differences between parent and mutant $H-2$ K glycoproteins from two H-2 K gene mutants: B6.C-H-2^{ba} (HZ1) and B6-H-2^{bd} (M505). J. Immunol. 118: 98.

37. Segall, M., F. H. Bach, M. L. Bach, J. L. Hussey, and D. T. Uehling. 1975. Correlation of MLC stimulation and clinical course in kdiney transplants. Transpl. Proc. VII, Supl. 1, pp. 41-43.

38. Widmer, M. B., B. J. Alter, F. H. Bach, M. L. Bach, and D. W. Bailey. 1973. Lymphocyte reactivity to serologically undetected components of the major histocompatibility complex. Nature New Biol. 242: 239.

39. Sopori, M., and F. H. Bach. 1979. Responses of thymocytes to alloantigenic stimuli. 13th International Leucocyte Culture Conference, Ottawa, Canada. Elsevier/North-Holland Biomedical Press, in press.

40. Wu, S., F. H. Bach, and M. Sopori. 1979. Differential allo-response of murine thymocytes to H-2 K region different recombinants and to H-2 K^b mutants. J. Immunol., submitted.

41. Isakov, N., B. Yankelevich, S. Segal, and M. Feldman. 1979. Differential immunogenic expression of an H-2-linked histocompatibility antigen on different tissues. Differences in survival between heart, thyroid and skin allografts. Transplant. 28: 31.

HLA and ocular disease

Robert B.Nussenblatt, M.D.

Clinical Branch, National Eye Institute, National Institutes of Health and Human Services, U.S. Department of Health, Education and Welfare, Bethesda, Maryland 20205

ABSTRACT

HLA typing has been widely employed in the field of ophthalmology. Four of the more rigorously HLA studied ocular entities are discussed here. Ankylosing spondylitis, though diagnosed purely on the basis of arthritic criteria, is known to have ocular disease associated with it in a high percentage of cases. The HLA B27 antigen is present in approximately 90% of Caucasians with this disease. However, the same association is considerably less striking in blacks, and that other HLA phenotype frequencies are also elevated. Recent reports suggest that the ocular disease may be a distinctly separate entity, with the B27 antigen being the common tie between the arthritic condition and the uveitis. Anterior uveitis in whites has been reported as having an HLA B27 association as well. This association appears to be the case only in those males with non-granulomatous, uniocular anterior segment disease, and many of those patients additionally manifest arthritic disease. HLA B27 was not found associated with acute recurrent iridocyclitis in Black Americans, but rather B5 and A1, suggesting an autoimmune etiology to this disease. Behcet's disease is a systemic ailment with frequently disastrous ocular complications. The strong association of HLA B5 and Behcet's disease in Japan has been well established. A less strong association of B5 with this disease has been reported in non-Japanese patients. The presumed ocular histoplasmosis syndrome is a major cause of visual impairment in the United States. It is the cause of legal blindness in approximately 1 out of 2000 individuals living in the Midwest region of the United States. An association of HLA B7 with those patients manifesting macular disease has been reported. No such association has been found in patients only manifesting peripheral retinal lesions.

Possible mechanisms by which HLA may play a role in ocular disease are discussed. On the basis of experimental work demonstrating a difference of susceptibility to the induction of uveitis in various histocompatible guinea pig strains, it is logical to assume that the same genetic variability to ocular inflammatory disease will be present amongst humans. Work showing that cell-mediated immune memory to the uveitogenic retinal S-antigen was present in sub-groups of many clinical uveitic entities would suggest that immune response genes "channel" immune responses in a predetermined way. The environmental role as it may interact with specific HLA phenotypes is supported by the geographic distribution of Behcet's disease and the presumed ocular histoplasmosis syndrome. A gene product closely associated with B27 has been demonstrated to cross react with Klebsiella pneumoniae antigens, thereby supporting the theory that molecular mimicry may be involved in the etiology of B27 positive patients with ankylosing spondylitis. It still though remains to be seen how exactly altered self, molecular mimicry, pathogen receptors, and immune response genes play a role in ocular disease processes.

INTRODUCTION

Vision is probably our most precious sense with references to ocular therapy mentioned by the Assyrians, Egyptians, and Greeks.[1] Perhaps of all sub-groups of disease entities in ophthalmology those that would fall under the category of ocular inflammatory disease remain the most difficult to treat, with their basic mechanisms still clouded. Sorsby[2] reported that ocular inflammatory disease (uveitis) was the cause of only 2.5% of the blind in England, but this figure rose to 8.3% when one only looked at the 30 - 39 year age group. In the United States,[3] it is estimated that uveitis is the cause of approximately 5% of legal blindness and 4.5% of severe visual impairment. The impact of HLA in ophthalmology as a tool for detection of disease susceptability and possible future regulation is most felt in the area of ocular inflammation. The four entities discussed in detail here will, I think, impress the reader as to the great variety in disease presenting to the ophthalmologist. These conditions have also been among the most vigorously studied for HLA associations. Their analyses should reveal the specific problems related to the study of eye diseases and where new techniques in immunogenetics will be best applied.

DISCUSSION

Ankylosing Spondylitis

Ankylosing spondylitis (AS) is a rheumatic disease that has become perhaps the "premier" HLA associated disease with ocular complications. The New York Criteria[4] for the diagnosis of ankylosing spondylitis are universally employed and eye disease is not mentioned. X-ray evidence of sacroiliitis is pre-eminent in the diagnosis. Diagnostic criteria also include limitation of motion of the lumbar spine in all three planes, history of lumbar pain, and limitation of chest expansion. In 1933, Kraupa[5] and Kunz[6] reported separately the association of this disease with iritis or anterior uveitis. The clinical characteristics of the ocular inflammation in AS is an unilateral non-granulomatous anterior segment response, occasionally involving both eyes at different times during the course of the disease. The disease is acute, i.e. pain, photophobia, and ciliary injection, with the inflammation lasting 3 - 5 weeks.[7] Early reports[8,9] made mention of this association, and stressed the need for iliosacral x-rays in the evaluation of patients with anterior uveitis. The incidence of uveitis with AS was first reported in 1937 by Schley[10], when he found 13.7% of 73 AS patients with anterior segment disease.

Investigators since then have reported a considerably higher percentage of eye involvement. Stanworth and Sharp[7] found evidence of past or active uveitis in 19% of 22 patients they studied. Interestingly, 2 patients reported that uveitis preceded joint pain or stiffness in the trunk or limbus by as long as four years. Wilkinson and Bywaters[11] studied 222 patients with 56 or 25% of them giving a history of uveitis. Uveitis arose within 10 years of the diagnosis of disease, and did not lead to band keratopathy. Only two patients in their study went on to develop "serious" visual impairment. This was approximately the same incidence reported by Bernstein et al[12] for those children with the diagnosis of juvenile AS, where the initial arthritic complaints are different than in adult onset AS. Both Stanworth and Sharp as well as Wilkinson and Bywaters stressed that there appeared to be no correlation between the activity of the arthritis and the ocular inflammation. Lenoch and colleagues'[13] large study of 635 cases showed an incidence of uveitis of 28.9% (179 cases). Those with AS were predominately male (570/625), and those with evidence of uveitis were as well (153/179). Haar[14] studied 358 "acute" and 169 chronic cases of anterior uveitis. Of the acute group, 40.9 has positive x-ray changes in the iliosacral region. Only one of the 169 patients in the chronic group manifested the same findings.

The difference in the incidence of AS in various races has been commented upon. Baum and Ziff[15] reported the rarity of AS in Black Americans, and epidemiologic studies[16] stress the essential non-existence of uveitis secondary to AS in Africa.

In the early 1970's, with more widespread use of HLA typing, Brewerton and colleagues[17], as well as other researchers,[18] reported a high association of HLA B27 in patients with AS. In Brewerton and colleagues' report, 72 of 75 Caucasian patients (96%) with advanced and easily diagnosable AS were identified as manifesting the B27 antigen while only 3 of 75 controls were found to have that phenotype. 21 of the patients studied had a history of uveitis. Additionally, 52% of first degree relatives were found to have B27 as well. Using tissue typing as a screening devise for the diagnosis of spondylitis, Cohen et al[19] reported that a high percentage of those males found to have B27 manifested typical arthritic and uveitic problems. They concluded that approximately 1 of 4 B27 positive white males were at risk for AS. New information has been recently added by Kemple et al's[20] study of HLA-D locus typing in AS. 44 patients with that disease were tested utilizing the one-way mixed leukocyte culture technique. No increased frequency of any Dw allele could be demonstrated in either the B27 positive or negative group.

The close association of B27 antigen and AS still leaves, upon close scrutiny, many unanswered questions. Clearly, in some "isolated" communities, such as the Pima Indians,[21] with a high incidence of the B27 antigen in the general population, there is the increased incidence of AS of 5.9% in this group as compared to 0.5% in the Caucasian community. On the other hand, while the incidence of AS in the Japanese is 4 in 10,000,[22] comparable to that found in American Caucasians, B27 is present in 1% of normal Japanese,[23] far below the incidence found in most Caucasian control groups reported in the literature. Khan[24] has shown that in addition to AS being three times less common in American Blacks than in whites, less than 60% of those blacks with AS are B27 positive, a ratio considerably below that found in studies with Caucasians. Khan et al[25] have also reported that in B27 negative Black AS patients, the incidence of the B7 CREG antigens were more than twice that found in B27 black controls (55.6 to 23.7%), thus suggesting that in blacks the B7 gene may be associated with the disease. And Duquenoy,[26] who was studying a small group of B27 negative white AS patients, found Cw1 and Cw2 in all cases, disputing the belief that AS is one of the few rigorously studied entities manifesting a histocompatibility association restricted to the B locus.

The question remains open as to whether the uveitis seen with AS may be an independent disease, and that the only link between the ocular and arthritic disorders is their common B27 association. Van der Linden et al's[27] report of 187 AS patients showed an incidence of uveitis in 21% of B27 positive and 12% of 27 negative patients. The difference was not thought to be significant. Khan et al,[28] though, found that 22 of 64 (34.9%) of their B27 positive AS patients had one or more episodes of uveitis, while only one of 15 (6.7%) of the B27 negative group gave that history. This disparity has been supported by Scharf and colleagues,[29] who found evidence of uveitis in 14 of 53 B27 positive patients, and in none of the 12 B27 negative patients that they studied.

Anterior Uveitis (iridocyclitis)

The designation "anterior uveitis" denotes both a clinical entity and the anatomic position of an ocular inflammatory response. Frequently, even after an extensive search for an underlying disease, the cause for the iridocyclitis remains elusive. The importance of diagnosing the underlying disease is self-evident. In addition, the ocular complications of an anterior uveitis such as glaucoma, band keratopathy, and cataract are serious threats to good vision.

The proposed pathogenesis for endogenous anterior uveitis is an immuno-

logic one. An experimental model described by Gamble et al[30] induced the
disease by immune complex formation. Alterations in vascular permeability
of the iris and ciliary body secondary to the immune complex deposition and
ensuing inflammation are thought to occur and leading thus to a breakdown
in the blood-aqueous barrier. Char et al[31] as well as others[32,33] have
reported the presence of circulating immune complexes in patients with
uveitis. According to Char et al, the immune complex appears to weigh approximately 2×10^6 daltons.

An association of HLA B27 and acute anterior uveitis was reported as
early as 1973 by Brewerton et al[34] with 26 of 50 patients bearing that antigen as opposed to 2 of 50 B27 positive controls. In that series, 29 of the
50 patients tested had no associated systemic disease, and only 8 of those 29
were B27 positive. Others, including Mapstone and Woodrow[35] and Zervas
et al,[36] confirmed the association of B27 with acute anterior uveitis in
Caucasians. On the other hand, Woodrow and colleagues[37] noted no increase
in the frequency of B27 in 10 patients with granulomatous uveitis that they
tested. The inflammatory response associated with B27 is described by all
the observers as that seen in AS; that is, non-granulomatous, unilateral,
and lasting for 3 - 4 weeks with serious complications being rare. Large
numbers of the patients reported were those with associated disease, not infrequently AS. The HLA association with chronic iridocyclitis in Caucasians
is less clear. Ehlers et al[38] found B27 not present in a large number of
Caucasians with chronic uveitis, but present in 71% of those with acute recurrent disease. Ohno and colleagues[39] found no increased incidence of B27
in those patients with the uveitis of rheumatoid arthritis or the chronic
iridocyclitis found in young girls. But Ohno et al[40] did find that the
incidence of B27 was statistically greater in 19 adult patients identified
as having a chronic anterior uveitis which was defined as painless, present
for greater than 6 months, and poorly responsive to medication.

Dr. K. Mittal and myself have recently typed 39 Black Americans with
acute recurrent iridocyclitis. None of the patients had any history of
rheumatologic disease (Table I). The phenotype frequency of B27 was not
found elevated in this patient group, whereas the B8 phenotype was 25.6%,
with control frequencies of that antigen being 6.7%. The A1 phenotype frequency was found to be elevated as well. Brewerton et al[41] reported that
A1 was present in 44% of 65 sarcoid patients with uveitis, with the HLA-B8
phenotype found elevated only in the sarcoid patients with arthritis. On
the basis of the association of the B8 loci with several auto-immune
entities,[42-44] this data would suggest that anterior uveitis, at least in

Table 1
SELECTED COMPARISONS OF THE HLA ANTIGEN FREQUENCIES IN
AMERICAN BLACKS WITH RECURRENT IRIDOCYCLITIS

Antigen	Phenotype Frequency (%)		'Exact' p	Relative Risk
	Controls (n=89)	Patients (n=39)		
HLA-A1	6.7	20.5	0.0310*	3.6
HLA-Aw24	2.3	12.8	0.0271*	6.4
HLA-B8	6.7	25.6	0.0067**	4.8
HLA-B27	6.7	7.7	1.0000	1.2
HLA-Bw39	1.1	10.3	0.0298*	10.1
HLA-Bw51	2.3	12.8	0.0271*	6.4

* p less than 0.05
** p less than 0.01

blacks, may be of a similar etiology.

Presumed Ocular Histoplasmosis Syndrome

Histoplasmosis capsulatum is a fungus found worldwide in many river valleys. It is endemic to the Midwestern region of the United States.[45] It is the rare cause of a systemic disease first described by Darling.[46] The systemic disease takes three major forms:[45] (1) an acute form with fever and x-ray evidence of pneumonitis which is usually not fatal, (2) an acute progressive form that is usually fatal in six weeks, and (3) a chronic progressive form similar in clinical appearance to tuberculosis.

The presumed ocular histoplasmosis syndrome is not a part of the entities briefly mentioned above. It is rather a characteristic choroiditis that, though reported previously, became more universally recognized with the report of Woods and Wahlen.[47] They theorized that lesions seen in the eye were due to a sub-clinical dissemination of the histoplasma organism. The pathologic reports of presumed cases[48,49] have shown lymphocytic infiltration of the choroid with overlying loss of retina and the retinal pigment epithelium. The term "presumed" remains an important feature to the name of this syndrome. To date, there has not been an incontrovertible histologic demonstration of the organism in a typical case of this disease. The significant lesion, though, is the maculopathy that strikes approximately one adult out of 1000 in endemic areas. The maculopathy is 1/6th as common in blacks,[50] but the response to histoplasmin skin testing is reported as being the same in both races.[51] Without therapy, 50% of those with the macular lesion will become legally blind in that eye.[52] Subretinal neovascularization leading to hemorrhage is the major complicating factor in macular disease of this entity.[53] Equally as important as the characteristic choroidal and retinal changes is that the vitreous remains clear; so that if inflammatory cells are visualized, a reassessment of the diagnosis of presumed ocular histoplasmosis must be made.[54]

HLA studies by Godfrey and associates[55] and Braley and associates[56] examined patients with "typical" peripheral lesions as well as with the maculopathy of presumed ocular histoplasmosis. 17 of 31 patients in one study and 14 out of 18 in the other demonstrated an association of HLA B7, with a phenotype frequency far exceeding that of controls and giving a relative risk value for the observed association in one study[56] of 11.8. Furthermore, in a report[57] looking at patients with only peripheral lesions, the B7 antigen frequency was 27% as compared to the control frequency for the antigen of 20% with the difference not statistically significant.

Clinical evidence of "typical" lesions still remains the foundation of the diagnosis in this entity. Both Schlaegel et al[50] and Krill et al[58] have reported series of "typical" cases where 11 and 9% respectively of patients had negative histoplasmin skin tests. Other disturbing features to this disease include 1) patients improve with corticosteroid therapy and not with amphotericin B, 2) Spaeth's review[59] of 134 proved cases of histoplasmosis revealing only 1 patient with typical ocular lesions, and 3) a similar ocular syndrome is seen in countries that are not endemic for histoplasmosis. HLA typing of patients from those non-endemic countries would be most informative in assessing the possible similarities or differences of these entities.

Behcet's Disease

Originally described by Professor Hulusi Behcet[60] as a triad of recurrent aphthous stomatitis, genital ulcers, and uveitis, this entity is a systemic disease affecting many organ systems. Skin manifestations are very common with erythema nodosum - like lesions, superficial thrombophlebitis, and acneiform or folliculitis-like lesions considered now as an integral part of the disease.[61] A curious hyperirritability of the skin seen in 60 - 70% of Behcet's patients was first reported by Jensen,[62] with induration and erythema arising 24 - 48 hours after a sterile needle prick, and often then becoming a pustule. In addition, polyarthritis, gastrointestinal disease, and large artery aneurysms have been reported.[63-65]

Central nervous system involvement is an ominous complication, and appears to be the main cause of death.[66] Inexact terminology in the literature in defining this entity has been troublesome. The unified diagnostic criteria as enumerated by the Japanese Research Committee of Behcet's Disease's Clinical Research Section presents the best concensus opinion.[67] A "complete" form of the disease is diagnosed only if the four major criteria of aphtha, skin, genital, and ocular lesions are present simultaneously or at different times during the course of the disease (Table 2).

The ocular manifestations of the disease, an anterior and/or posterior uveitis, are the most serious of the major criteria. An intense anterior uveitis with hypopyon is one of the hallmarks of the disease. Posteriorly, the superficial and deep layers of the retina are involved, with the most intense areas of inflammation found around the retinal vessels. There is as well an accompanying choroiditis and/or choriocapillaritis. The periphlebitis of the retinal vessels is frequently associated with a vitritis as well as recurrent vitreal hemorrhages.[68] Exacerbations of the ocular component are common with an average span from onset to ultimate blindness in untreated cases being calculated as 3.4 years.[69] Therapy with immuno-suppressives, particularly chlorambucil, appears to have favorably changed this statistic significantly.[66,70]

Behcet's disease occurs most frequently in Japan and the Mediterranean basin.[71] In Japan, the disease makes up 25% of all endogenous uveitis cases seen,[72] and accounts for 12% of blindness in the young-middle aged adult groups in that country.[73] In a survey of 7,000 Japanese hospitals[74] Behcet's disease was found to be more prevalent in the northern districts of the country, suggesting a possible environmental role. An overall estimate of

TABLE 2

Guidelines for the Diagnosis of Behcet's Disease

Complete Type:	Four Major Criteria, i.e.
	aphthous ulceration, skin genital, and ocular lesions
Incomplete :	1) Three Major Criteria
	2) Ocular lesions plus one other major criterion
Suspect :	Two Major Criteria
Possible :	One of the Major Criteria
All lesions can occur simultaneously or at different times during the course of the disease.	
Adapted from: Editorial, Jpn. J. Ophthalmol. 18:291, 1974.	

the prevalence of the disease was calculated as 7.0-8.5/100,000 citizens. In Japan, complete Behcet's was more common amongst males, with a familial occurrence of 2.1%.

The figures are strikingly different for the United States. In a survey of 5,500 consecutive cases of uveitis seen at the Uveitis Survey Clinic of the University of California at San Francisco,[75] some 22 patients with complete or incomplete Behcet's were identified. Only 7 cases were diagnosed out of 1,700 cases of uveitis at the Institute of Ophthalmology in London.[76]

A significant advance in understanding the underlying pathology of Behcet's has been the finding of the high incidence of HLA B5 in patients with this disease. In three separate studies,[77-79] Ohno and colleagues have repeatedly demonstrated the presence of B5 in 60-75% of Japanese patients with the disease while control phenotype frequencies range around 28%. Ohno et al[79] concluded that, in Japan, B5 was most commonly found amongst males with the complete form, and least commonly found amongst women with the incomplete form not having ocular lesions. In studying a small group of Americans with this disease, Ohno and co-workers[75] reported that only 1 of the 6 Caucasians, but 2 of the 5 orientals tested were B5 positive. Interestingly, the 2 Caucasian patients who manifested the complete form of the disease were B5 negative. O'Duffy et al[80] failed to find any HLA antigens in greater frequency in their 26 patients studied at the Mayo Clinic. Other studies,[81-83] though, have demonstrated a close association of B5 with the disease in Caucasian patients, supporting a universal role for this antigen in Behcet's disease.

The etiology and the role of the B5 antigen in the disease process remains a mystery. Exogenous, environmental factors may play a significant role in the expression of this disease. There has been an enormous increase in the incidence of the disease in Japan since World War Two.[84] Most interestingly, no Japanese Americans living in Hawaii have been reported to have the disease.[85] Tubular structures suggestive of the nucleocapsid of a myovirus have been described in the retina and uvea of eyes from Behcet's patients that have been histologically studied.[86] However, Tokuda and Uyama[87] were unable to demonstrate high anti-viral titers in the serum of Behcet's disease patients. The discovery of the major factors in the etiology of this potentially devastating disease still awaits us.

Other Ocular Diseases

Various ocular entities have been scrutinized with the use of HLA typing and their results summarized elsewhere.[88] A thorough review of all of them is not within the scope of this report. Significant non-correlations

TABLE 3

Summary of HLA Studies

Disease	Author(s) and Reference Number	Increase in Phenotype Frequency
Ankylosing Spondylitis	Brewerton et al (17)	B27 in Caucasians
	Cohen et al (19)	B27 in Caucasians
	Kemple et al (20)	No increase in Dw allele
	Schlosstein et al (18)	B27 in Caucasians
	Khan et al (24)	B27 in Blacks, lower incidence
	Khan et al (25)	B7 in B27 neg Blacks
	Duquenoy (26)	Cw1, Cw2 in B27 neg Whites.
	Van der Linden et al (27)	Uveitis in B27 positive and negative group
	Khan et al (28)	Uveitis in B27 group only
	Scharf et al (29)	Uveitis in B27 group only
Anterior Uveitis	Brewerton et al (34)	B27 in Caucasians
	Mapstone and Woodrow (35)	B27 in Caucasians
	Zervas et al (36)	B27 in Caucasians
	Woodrow et al (37)	None in granulomatous uveitis
	Ehlers et al (38)	None in chronic uveitis
		B27 in acute recurrent uveitis
	Ohno et al (39)	None in uveitis of rheumatoid arthritis
		None in chronic iridocyclitis of young girls
	Nussenblatt and Mittal (In Preparation)	B8 Al in American Blacks with acute recurrent iridocyclitis

Presumed Ocular Histoplasmosis Syndrome	Godfrey et al (55)	B7 Patients with macular disease
	Braley et al (56)	B7 Patients with macular disease
	Meredith et al (57)	None, Patients with peripheral retinal
Behcet's Disease	Ohno et al (77 – 79)	B5 in Japanese patients
	Ohno et al (75)	None in American patients
	O'Duffy et al (80)	None in American patients
	Rosselet et al (81)	B5 in Europeans
	Godeau et al (82)	B5 in Europeans
	Bloch-Michel et al (83)	B5 in Europeans

should be mentioned. Though earlier reports suggested an HLA correlation with the pigment dispersion syndrome and open angle glaucoma,[89,90] several more recent reports have failed to support these original suppositions.[91,92,93] Based on the already vast animal and substantial human studies, it would seem that HLA typing will remain most fruitfully utilized in the study of ocular diseases with a proposed inflammatory or immune auto-regulatory component.

Possible Mechanisms

The exact mechanisms by which HLA might play a role in human disease remains speculative. A variety of possible theories have been proposed;[94,95] those frequently cited include: 1) The HLA genes are closely linked to the immune response genes involved in the pathogenic process. 2) The altered self theory in which viruses alter antigens coded for by the D retion thereby permitting autoimmunity. 3) The receptor theory, in which certain HLA phenotypes serve as a receptacle for a pathologic virus or other antigen, therefore making the cell surface susceptible to a specific disease and 4) The molecular mimicry theory in which the histocompatibility antigen shares antigenic determinants with a pathogen, thereby leading to a tolerance to the invading organism. It could be that various histocompatibility phenotypes may participate in very different immune mechanisms. The diseases reviewed here all have significant associations with HLA phenotypes that are not always identical (Table 3). Guinea pig strain variations in the susceptibility to the induction of experimental allergic uveitis is well known.[96] Induction of the disease in the histocompatible strain 13 can be achieved, while the strain 2 guinea pigs remain resistant. This demonstration of variability in ocular inflammatory disease thus provides a theoretical basis for the assumption that genetic factors play a role in the susceptibility of humans to ocular inflammatory diseases.

Cell mediated immunity has been shown to be important in experimental uveitis.[97,98] We[99] have reported evidence of cell mediated immune recognition to the S-antigen in uveitis patients. The S-antigen is a retinal specific uveitogenic antigen found in mammals capable of inducing ocular inflammation with immunizing doses as low as 5µg.[100] The in vitro anamnestic response to the S-antigen was not restricted to a specific ocular entity, but rather sub-groups of patients from various uveitic entities manifested this response. It is tempting to speculate that immune response genes are pre-determined systems by which responses are "channelled". Therefore, similar immune pathways may be followed in different ocular inflammatory conditions depending upon the gene phenotypes.

The relationship of HLA to suppressor cell function is just beginning to unfold. This area is of potentially great importance in uveitis, where recurrences pose such a great problem. An adherant suppressor cell has been reported in patients with herpes keratitis,[101] perhaps playing a role in chronic cases. Zilko and colleagues[102] reported impaired cell suppressor functions in myasthenia gravis patients with B8. A suppressor cell defect in inflammatory bowel disease has also been reported;[103] this being, as uveitis, a localized nidus of disease of presumed immune origin.

The role of the environment and HLA is of tremendous interest in ocular inflammatory disease. Ankylosing spondylitis patients have been shown to have Klebsiella pneumoniae in their feces more frequently than in the control population,[103] and evidence now indicates that a gene product closely associated with B27 may cross react with certain Klebsiella products.[104] Behcet's disease has such a well defined epidemiologic distribution that one cannot but assume that environmental factors play a role. The distribution of the presumed ocular histoplasmosis syndrome also suggests this.

HLA has a well deserved place in ocular immunology, with its development providing an important addition to the characterization of disease entities and giving some insight into pathogenesis. But it still remains to be seen how exactly altered self, molecular mimicry, pathogen receptors, and immune response genes plays a role in ocular disease processes.

Acknowledgements

I thank Dr. Igal Gery for his helpful comments, and Mrs. Joan Lee for her technical assistance.

REFERENCES

1.   Duke-Elder, S. 1962. System of Ophthalmology. The Foundations of Ophthalmology, Vol. VII. Henry Kimpton, London. Pp. 464-466.
2.   Sorbsy, A. 1956. Causes of blindness in England. 1951-54. Her Majesty's Stationary Office, London. Pp. 6-37.
3.   U.S., DHEW: DHS:, NIH. 1976. Interim Report of the National Advisory Eye Council, Support for Vision Research. Pp. 20-22.
4.   Bennett, P.H., and P.H.N. Wood (ed.). 1968. Population Studies of the Rheumatic Diseases. Excerpta Medica Foundation, Amsterdam. Pp. 456-457.
5.   Kraupa, E. 1933. Iritis und "spondylarthritis ankylopoetica". Klin. Monatsbl. Augenheilkd. 91:493.
6.   Kunz, E. 1933. Ueber das Vorkommen von Iritis beichronisch-entzündlicher Wirbelsäuleversteifung (Spondylarthritis ankylopoetica). Klin. Monatsbl. Augenheilkd. 91:153.
7.   Stanworth, A., and J. Sharp. 1956. Uveitis and rheumatic diseases. Ann. Rheum. Dis. 15:140.
8.   Franceschetti, A. 1946. Les affections oculaires d'origine rheumatismale. Ophthalmologica 111:242.

9. Hogan, M.J., S.J. Kimura, and P. Thygescn. 1957. Uveitis in association with rheumatism. A.M.A. Arch. Ophthalmol. 57:400.

10. Schley, H. 1937. Spondylarthritis ankylopoetica bei iritis. Klin. Monatsbl. Augenheilkd. 98:780.

11. Wilkinson, M., and E.G.L. Bywaters. 1958. Clinical features and cause of ankylosing spondylitis. Ann. Rheum. Dis. 17:209.

12. Bernstein, B.H., B.H. Singsen, A. Lorber, H.K. Kornreich, K.K. King, and V. Hanson. 1979. Juvenile ankylosing spondylitis: are adult criteria appropriate? Arthritis Rheum. 22:593.

13. Lenoch, F., V. Kralik, and J. Bartos. 1959. "Rheumatic" iritis and iridocyclitis. Ann. Rheum. Dis. 18:45.

14. Haar, M. 1960. Rheumatic iridocyclitis. Acta. Ophthalmol. 38:37.

15. Baum, J., and M. Ziff. 1970. The rarity of ankylosing spondylitis in the Black race. Arthritis Rheum. 13:305.

16. Perkins, E.S. 1976. Symposium on Uveitis. Epidemiology of Uveitis. Trans. Ophthalmol. Soc. U.K. 96:105.

17. Brewerton, D.A., F.D. Hart, A. Nicholls, M. Caffrey, D.C.O. James, and R.D. Sturrock. 1973. Ankylosing spondylitis and HL-A 27. Lancet 1:904.

18. Schlosstein, L., P.I. Terasaki, R. Bluestone, and C. Pearson. 1973. High association of an HL-A antigen - W27, with ankylosing spondylitis. N. Engl. J. Med. 288:704.

19. Cohen, L.M., K.K. Mittal, F.R. Schmid, L.F. Rogers, and K.L. Cohen. 1976. Increased risk for spondylitis stigmata in apparently healthy HL-Aw27 Men. Ann. Intern. Med. 84:1.

20. Kemple, K., R.A. Gatti, W. Leibold, J. Klinenberg, and R. Bluestone. 1979. HLA-D locus typing in ankylosing spondylitis and Reiter's syndrome. Arthritis Rheum. 22:371.

21. Pees, E.K., D.D. Kostyu, R.C. Elston, and D.B. Amos. 1972. HLA profiles of the Pima Indians of Arizona. In Histocompatibility Testing 1972. Edited by J. Dausset and J. Colombani. Munksgaard, Copenhagen. Pp. 345-349.

22. Tsujimoto, M. 1970. The frequency of ankylosing spondylitis and its diagnostic criteria. Orthop. Surg. (Japan) 5:514.

23. Mittal, K.K., T. Haseguawa, A. Ting, M.R. Mickey, and P.I. Terasaki. 1972. Genetic variation in the HL-A system between Anius, Japanese, and Caucasians. Histocompatibility Testing. 1972. Munksgaard, Copenhagen Pp. 187-195.

24. Khan, M.A. 1978. Race-related differences in HLA association with ankylosing spondylitis and Reiter's Disease in American Blacks and Whites. J. Natl. Med. Assoc. 70:41.

25. Khan, M.A., I. Kushner, W.E. Braun, B.Z. Schacter, and A.G. Steinberg. 1977. HLA-B7 and ankylosing spondylitis in American Blacks. N. Engl. J. Med. 297:513.

26. Duquesnoy, R.J., F. Kozin, and G.E. Rodey. 1978. High prevalence of HLA-B27, Cwl, and Cw2 in patients with seronegative spondyloarthritis. Tissue Antigens 12:58.

27. Van der Linden, J.M., K. de Ceulaer, L.K. van Romunde, and A. Cats. 1977. Ankylosing spondylitis without HLA B27. J. Rheumatol. (Suppl. 3) 4:56.

28. Khan, M.A., I. Kushner, and W.E. Braun. 1977. Comparison of clinical features in HLA B27 positive and negative patients with ankylosing spondylitis. Arthritis Rheum. 20:909.

29. Scharf, J., M. Nahir, J. Scharf, R. Brick, O. Gidoni, A. Barzilai, and S. Zonis. 1979. Anterior uveitis in ankylosing spondylitis: a histocompatibility study. Ann. Ophthalmol. 11:1061.

30. Gamble, C.N., S.B. Arnson, and F.B. Brescia. 1970. The pathogenesis of recurrent immunologic (Auer) uveitis. Arch. Ophthalmol. 84:331.

31. Char, D.H., P. Stein, R. Masi, and M. Christensen. 1979. Immune complexes in uveitis. Am. J. Ophthalmol. 87:678.

32. Rahi, A.H.S., E.J. Holborow, E.S. Perkins, and W.J. Dinning. 1979. What is endogenous uveitis. In Immunology and Immunopathology of the Eye. Edited by A.M. Silverstein and G.R. O'connoer. Masson Publishing USA, Inc. New York. Pp. 23-28.

33. Dernouchamps, J.P., and J. Michiels. 1979. Circulating antigen-antibody complexes in the aqueous humor. In Immunology and Immunopathology of the Eye. Edited by A.M. Silverstein and G.R. O'Connor. Masson Publishing USA, Inc. New York. Pp. 40-45.

34. Brewerton, D.A., M. Caffrey, A. Nicholls, D. Walters, and D.C.O. James. 1973. Acute anterior uveitis and HL-A27. Lancet 2:994.

35. Mapstone, R., and J.C. Woodrow. 1975. HL-A27 and acute anterior uveitis. Br. J. Ophthalmol. 59:270.

36. Zervas, J., G. Tsokos, G. Papadakis, E. Kabouklis, and D. Papadopoulos. 1977. HLA-B27 frequency in Greek patients with acute anterior uveitis. Br. J. Ophthalmol. 61:699.

37. Woodrow, J.C., R. Mapstone, J. Anderson, and N. Usher. 1975. HL-A27 and anterior uveitis. Tissue Antigens 6:116.

38. Ehlers, N., F. Kissmeyer-Nielsen, K.E. Kjerbye, and L.U. Lamm. 1974. HL-A27 in acute and chronic uveitis. Lancet 1:99.

39. Ohno, S., D.H. Char, S.J. Kimura, and G.R. O'Connor. 1977. HLA antigens and antinuclear antibody titers in juvenile chronic iridocyclitis. Br. J. Ophthalmol. 61:59.

40. Ohno, S., S.J. Kimura, G.R. O'Connor, and D.H. Char. 1977. HLA antigens and uveitis. Br. J. Ophthalmol. 61:62.

41. Brewerton, D.A., C. Cockburn, D.C.O. James, D.G. James, and E. Neville. 1977. HLA antigens in sarcoidosis. Clin. Exp. Immunol. 27:277.

42. Grumet, F.C., A. Coukell, and J.G. Bodmer. 1971. Histocompatibility (HL-A) antigens associated with systemic lupus erythematosus: a possible genetic predisposition to disease. N. Engl. J. Med. 285:193.

43. Irvine, W.J., R.S. Gray, P.J. Morris, and A. Ting. 1977. Correlation of HLA and thyroid antibodies with clinical course of thyrotoxicosis treated with antithyroid drugs. Lancet 2:298.

44. Behan, P.O., J.A. Simpson, and H. Dicke. 1973. Immune response genes in myasthenia gravis. Lancet 2:1033.

45. Asbury, T. 1966. The status of presumed ocular histoplasmosis: Including a report of a survey. Trans. Am. Ophthalmol. Soc. 64:371.

46. Darling, S.T. 1906. A protozoan general infection producing pseudotubules in lungs and focal necrosis in the liver, spleen, and lymph nodes. JAMA 46:1283.

47. Woods, A.C., and H.E. Wahlen. 1960. The probable role of benign histoplasmosis in the etiology of granulomatous uveitis. Am. J. Ophthalmol. 49:205.

48. Makley, T.A., E.L. Craig, and S.W. Long. 1977. Histopathology of presumed ocular histoplasmosis. Palestra Oftalmologica Panamericana 1:71.

49. Meredith, T.A., W.R. Green, S.N. Key III, G.S. Dolin, and A.E. Maumenee. 1977. Ocular histoplasmosis: Clinicopathologic correlation of 3 cases. Surv. Ophthalmol. 22:189.

50. Schlaegel, T.F., J.C. Weber, E. Helveston, and D. Kennedy. 1967. Presumed histoplasmic choroiditis. Am. J. Ophthalmol. 63:919.

51. Ziedberg, L.D. 1956. The microdistribution of histoplasmin sensitivity in an endemic area. In Proceedings of the Conference on Histoplasmosis. 1952. Edited by M.J. Willis. Public Health Monograph 39. Pp. 190-197.

52. Schlaegel, T.F. 1977. Ocular histoplasmosis. Gruna and Stratton, New York. P. XIII.

53. Ibid., p. 53

54. Ibid., Pp. 56-58.

55. Godfrey, W.A., R. Sabates, and D.E. Cross. 1978. Association of presumed ocular histoplasmosis with HLA-B7. Am. J. Ophthalmol. 85:854.

56. Braley, R.E., T.A. Meredith, T.M. Aaberg, S.M. Koethe, and J.A. Witkowski. 1978. The prevalence of HLA-B7 in presumed ocular histoplasmosis. Am. J. Ophthalmol. 85:859.
57. Meredith, T.A., R.E. Smith, R.E. Braley, J.A. Witkowski, and S.M. Koethe. 1978. The prevalence of HLA-B7 in presumed ocular histoplasmosis in patients with peripheral atrophic scars. Am. J. Ophthalmol. 86:325.
58. Krill, A.E., M.I. Chishti, B.A. Klein, F.W. Newell, and A.M. Potts. 1969. Multifocal inner choroiditis. Trans. Am. Acad. Ophthalmol. Otolaryngol. 73:222.
59. Spaeth, G.L. 1967. Absence of so-called histoplasma uveitis in 134 cases of proven histoplasmosis. Arch. Ophthalmol. 77:41.
60. Behcet, H. 1937. Über rezidivierende aphthose durch ein virus verursachte Geschwure am Mund, am Auge, und an der Genitalen. Derm. Wschr. 105:1152.
61. Shimizu, T. 1979. Clinicopathological Studies on Behcet's Disease. In Behcet's Disease. Proceedings of an International Symposium on Behcet's Disease. Istanbul, 29-30 September 1977. Edited by N. Dilsen, M. Konice, and C. Övül. Excerpta Medica, Amsterdam. Pp. 9-43.
62. Jensen, T. 1941. Sur les ulcérations aphtheuses la mugueuse de la bouche et de la peau génitale combinee avec les symptôms (Syndrome de Behcet). Acta Dermat. Vener. 22:64.
63. Dilsen, N., M. Konice, and C. Övül. 1979. Arthritic patterns in Behcet's disease. 1979. In Behcet's Disease. Proceedings of an International Symposium on Behcet's Disease, Istanbul, 29-30 September 1977. Edited by N. Dilsen, M. Konice, and C. Övül. Excerpta Medica, Amsterdam. Pp. 145-155.
64. Boe, J., J.B. Dalgaard, and D. Scott. 1958. Mucocutaneous-ocular syndrome with intestinal involvement; a clinical and pathologic study of four fatal cases. Am. J. Med. 25:857.
65. Enoch, B.A., J.L. Castillo-Olivares, T.C.L. Khoo, R.G. Grainger, and L. Henry. 1968. Major Vascular Complications in Behcet's Syndrome. Postgrad. Med. J. 44:453.
66. O'Duffy, J.D. 1979. Prognosis in Behcet's Syndrome. In Behcet's Disease. Proceedings of an International Symposium on Behcet's Disease, Istanbul, 29-30 September 1977. Edited by N. Dilsen, M. Konice, and C. Övül. Excerpta Medica, Amsterdam. Pp. 191-198.
67. Editorial: Behcet's Disease. 1974. Jpn. J. Ophthalmol. 18:291.
68. BenEzra, D., and R.B. Nussenblatt. 1978. Ocular manifestations of Behcet's disease. J. Oral. Path. 7:431.
69. Mamo. J.G. 1970. The rate of visual loss in Behcet's disease. Arch. Ophthalmol. 84:851.
70. Mamo, J.G., and S.A. Azzam. 1970. Treatment of Behcet's disease with chlorambucil. Arch. Ophthalmol. 84: 446.
71. Bietti, G.B., and F. Bruna. 1966. An Ophthalmic Report on Behcet's Disease. In Behcet's Disease. Edited by M. Monacelli and P. Nazzaro. Karger, Basel. Pp. 79-110.
72. Araki, Y. 1971. Classified Incidence of Uveitis (1965-1969). Acta Soc. Ophthalmol. Jap. 75:389.
73. Shimizu. T., I. Tanaka, and T. Ogino. 1971. Behcet's disease in Japan. Igaku no Ayumi. 75:332.
74. Yamamoto, S., H. Toyokawa, J. Matsubara, H. Yanai, Y. Inaba, K. Nakae, and M. Ono. 1974. A Nation-Wide Survey of Behcet's Disease in Japan. Jpn. J. Ophthalmol. 18:282.
75. Ohno, S., D.H. Char, S.J. Kimura, and G.R. O'Connor. 1978. Studies on HLA Antigens in American Patients with Behcet's Disease. Jpn. J. Ophthalmol. 22:58.
76. Perkins, E.S. 1961. Discussion on Behcet's Disease. Ophthalmological Aspects. Proc. Roy. Soc. Med. 54:106.
77. Ohno, S., E. Nakayama, S. Sugiura, K. Itakura, K. Aoki, and M. Aizawa.

1975. Specific histocompatibility antigens associated with Behcet's disease. Am. J. Ophthalmol. 80:636.

78. Ohno, S., S. Sugiura, K. Itakura, and M. Aizawa. 1978. Further studies on HLA antigens in Behcet's disease. Jpn. J. Ophthalmol. 22:62.

79. Ohno, S., S. Sugiura, M. Ohguchi, and K. Aoki. 1979. Close association of HLA-B5 with Behcet's disease. In Immunology and Immunopathology of the Eye. Edited by A.M. Silverstein and G.R. O'Connor. Masson Publishing USA, Inc, New York. Pp. 15-17.

80. O'Duffy, J.D., H.F. Taswell, and L.R. Elveback. 1976. HL-A antigens in Behcet's disease. J. Rheumatol. 3:1.

81. Rosselet, E., W.M. Saudan, and M. Jeannet. 1976. Recherche des antigenes HLA dans la maladie de Behcet. Ophthalmologica. 172:116.

82. Godeau, P., D. Torre, R. Campinchi, E. Bloch-Michel, M. Schmid, A. Nunez-Roldan, J. Hors, and J. Dausset. 1976. HLA--5 and Behcet's disease. In HLA and Disease. Edited by J. Dausset and A. Svejgaard. INSERM, Paris. P. 101.

83. Bloch-Michel, E., R. Campinchi, J.Y. Muller, M. Binaghi, and J. Sales. 1979. HLA antigens and uveitis with special reference to Behcet's disease, chronic herpes simplex, toxoplasmosis, and recurrent anterior uveitis. In Immunology and Immunopathology of the Eye. Edited by A.M. Silverstein and G.R. O'Connor. Masson Publishing USA, Inc. New York. Pp. 10-14.

84. Shimizu, K., S. Ishikawa, M. Miyata, H. Yoshida, and H. Kubo. 1979. Relationships between the changes of serum copper levels and ocular attacks in Behcet's disease (an etiological consideration). In Behcet's Disease. Proceedings of an International Symposium on Behcet's Disease. Istanbul, 29-30 September, 1977. Edited by N. Dilsen, M. Konice, and C. Övül. Excerpta Medica, Amsterdam. Pp. 61-65.

85. Hirohato. T., M. Kuratsune, A. Nomura, and S. Jimi. 1975. Prevalence of Behcet's syndrome in Hawaii. Hawaii Med. J. 34:244.

86. Sugiura, S., H. Matsuda, K. Aripa, M. Igarashi, and M. Kisoh. 1974. Electron microscopy of the retina and uvea in Behcet's disease. Nippon Ganka Gakkai Zasshi. 78:394.

87. Tokuda, M., and M. Uyama. 1975. Virological study on etiology of Behcet's disease. Studies on the etiology, treatment, and prevention on Behcet's disease in 1974. In the 1975 Annual Report of Behcet's Disease Research Committee of Japan, Ministry of Health and Welfare. Pp. 35-41.

88. Rahi, A.H.S. 1979. HLA and eye disease. Br. J. Ophthalmol. 63:283.

89. Becker, B. D. Shin, D.G. Cooper, and M.A. Kass. 1977. The pigment dispersion syndrome. Am. J. Ophthalmol. 83:161.

90. Shin, D.H., B. Becker, and S.R. Waltman. 1977. The prevalence of HLA-B12 and HLA-B7 antigens in POAG. Arch. Ophthalmol. 95:224.

91. Grabner, G., and W.R. Mayr. 1979. HLA antigens and primary open-angle glaucoma. In Immunology and Immunopathology of the Eye. Edited by A.M. Silverstein and G.R. O'Connor. Masson Publishing USA, Inc. New York. Pp. 18-22.

92. David, R., G. Maier, I. Baumgarten, and C. Abrahams. 1979. HLA antigens in glaucoma and ocular hypertension. Br. J. Ophthalmol. 63:293.

93. Kaiser-Kupfer, M.I. and K.K. Mittal. 1978. The HLA and ABO antigens in pigment dispersion syndrome. Am. J. Ophthalmol. 85:368.

94. Zinkernagel, R.M., and P.C. Doherty. 1977. Possible mechanisms of disease-susceptibility association with major transplantation antigens. In HLA and Disease. Edited by J. Dausset and A. Svejgaard. Williams and Wilkins Co. Baltimore. Pp. 256-268.

95. Amos, D.B., and F.E. Ward. 1977. Theoretical consideration in the association between HLA and disease. In HLA and Disease. Edited by J. Dausset and A. Svejgaard. Williams and Wilkins Co. Baltimore. Pp. 269-279.

96. McMaster, P.R.B., V.G. Wong, and J.D. Owens. 1976. The propensity of different strains of guinea pigs to develop experimental autoimmune uveitis.

Mod. Probl. Ophthalmol. 16:62.

97. de Kozak, Y, W.S. Youn, M. Bogossian, and J.P. Faure. 1976. Humoral and cellular immunity to retinal antigens in guinea pigs. Mod. Probl. Ophthalmol. 16:51.

98. Ticho, U., A.M. Silverstein, and G.A. Cole. 1974. Immunopathogenesis of LCM virus-induced uveitis: the role of T lymphocytes. Invest. Ophthalmol. 13:229.

99. Nussenblatt. R., I. Gery, E.J. Ballintine, and W.B. Wacker. Cellular immune responsiveness of uveitis patients to retinal S-antigen. Am. J. Ophthalmol. (in press).

100. Wacker, W.B., L.A. Donoso, C.M. Kalsow, J.A. Yankeelov Jr., and D.T. Organisciak. 1977. Experimental allergic uveitis. Isolation, characterization, and localization of a soluble uveitopathogenic antigen from Bovine retina. J. Immunol. 119:1949.

101. Lopez, C., R. Ryshke, and S. Bloomfield. 1978. Adherent suppressor cells in patients with deep stromal disease associated with herpes keratitis. In Proc. Assoc. Res. Vision Ophthalmol., Spring Meeting, Sarasota, Florida. P. 273.

102. Zilko, P.J., R.L. Dawkins, K. Holmes, and C. Witt. 1979. Genetic control of suppressor lymphocyte function in myasthenia gravis: Relationship of impaired suppressor function to HLA-B8/DRw3 and cold reactive lymphocytotoxic antibodies. Clin. Immunol. Immunopathol. 14:222.

103. Hodgson, H.J.F., J.R. Wands, and K.J. Isselbacher. 1978. Decreased suppressor cell activity in inflammatory bowel disease. Clin. Exp. Immunol. 32:451.

104. Ebringer, R.W., D.R. Cawdell, P. Cowling, and A. Ebringer. 1978. Sequential studies in ankylosing spondylitis. Association of Klebsiella pneumoniae with active disease. Ann. Rheum. Dis. 37:146.

105. Seager, K., H.V. Bashir, A.F. Geczy, J. Edmonds, and A. de Vere-Tyndell. 1979. Evidence for a specific B27-associated cell surface marker on lymphocytes of patients with ankylosing spondylitis. Nature 277:68.

The current status of associations between major abnormalities of HLA antigen frequency and disease

Warren Strober, M.D.

Head, Immunophysiology Section, Metabolism Branch, National Cancer Institute, National Institutes of Health

Introduction

Diseases associated with particular HLA specificities are generally similar in that they are diseases of unknown etiology, and are caused or influenced by poorly defined genetic and/or environmental factors. In addition, the HLA-associated diseases tend to be chronic and in the great majority of cases, they are associated with immunologic abnormalities. As indicated by Dausset, these diseases can be grouped into several large categories based on the main HLA gene or locus that is affected[1]. The largest category consists of those diseases associated with HLA-D locus and/or HLA-B locus abnormalities. These diseases have in common numerous "autoimmune" manifestations including the presence of organ specific antibodies, high titers of anti-viral antibodies -sometimes suggesting a viral etiology, female predominance, and a hereditary pattern suggesting polygenic inheritance. The most striking and remarkable association in this category is the association between a large number of autoimmune diseases (or, more precisely, diseases characterized by immunologic abnormalities) with an increased frequency of either HLA-B8 and HLA-Dw3 or HLA-B7 and HLA-Dw2. This association between a restricted HLA genotype and a large number of different diseases of widely varying phenotype is suggestive of the presence of a common pathophysiologic mechanism which is acting in conjunction with a variety of independent genetic and environmental factors to produce unique disease entities.

Another category of HLA-associated diseases consists of the group of diseases in which the frequency of a particular HLA-B locus antigen, HLA-B27 is increased. This category includes ankylosing spondylitis in which HLA-B27 occurs in almost 90% of cases, as well as several other arthropathies. This category also includes a number of diseases suchas inflammatory bowel diseases, dysenteries caused by Salmonella, Shigella and Yersinia organisms, as well as "non-specific" urethritis and conjuncti-vitis, which are not themselves marked by an increased frequency of HLA-B27 yet are frequently associated with conditions such as ankylosing spondylitis or Reiter's syndrome which are so characterized. Careful study of this situation reveals that HLA-B27 does in fact occur quite often in the sub-set of patients with these diseases who display the associated conditions (ankylosing spondylitis or Reiter's syndrome) and HLA-B27 thus appears to be a genetic factor that leads to particular associated clinical condition when other, non-HLA-B27 related, diseases occur.

The final category of diseases associated with particular HLA genes are diseases caused by defects in genes lying close to the major histocom-patibility region but which are themselves not part of the major histo-compatibility (MHC) complex, i.e., genes not coding for HLA antigens. C2 deficiency and 21-hydroxylase deficiency presumably caused by mutations in the genes controlling the synthesis of C2 and 21-hydroxylase respectively and which lie in the midst of the MHC are examples of diseases in this category[2,3]. The defects in these cases show clear-cut genetic influence, with almost total penetrance and no sex predominance.

Not included in any of these categories are a variety of diseases which cannot be classified in any way, and must therefore be considered under "miscellaneous" HLA-disease associations (see Table II). These associations involve a wide variety of HLA antigens and underscore the point that the HLA genes are likely to play a wide variety of roles in the causation of disease.

As we shall see, in most (if not all) instances, it is not the HLA genes coding for A,B,C or D locus antigens that are considered to be directly involved in disease processes, but rather the genes in the major histocompatibility locus that are in linkage disequilibrium with the HLA genes. By linkage disequilibrium we refer to the fact that certain sets of genes in the HLA locus tend to occur together in the same individual far more frequently than one would expect if one assumed that crossover events are occuring at random frequency at any point in the HLA linkage group. Thus, HLA-B8 occurs along with HLA-Dw3 in the same individual more frequently than one would predict from the individual frequency of these specificities. In a similar way, it is possible that a "disease gene" occurs along with both HLA-B8 and HLA-Dw3 more frequently than one would expect by chance, thus giving rise to the association between a disease and a given HLA specificity. Linkage disequilibrium may occur for any of a variety of reasons, but the most intriguing (and also the most likely) is that certain sets of HLA genes constitute a "supergene" whose components are mutually necessary for certain functions and which provide a selective advantage to the organism (vide supra). This implies that the HLA genes already identified as being associated with certain diseases should probably not be regarded only as marker genes, but rather as participants in the disease process.

In the discussion to follow we will review first the evidence relative to the association between HLA antigens with a variety of diseases, first those diseases associated with HLA-B8 and HLA-Dw3, followed by those associated with other B and D locus antigens. We will then consider, in a more general way, the mechanisms whereby HLA-associated genes could have a bearing on the diseases in question, particularly insofar as such genes affect individuals with these diseases in a common and/or universal manner.

Individual Diseases Associated with HLA-B8 and HLA-Dw3 (HLA-B8/Dw3).
All of the diseases comprising the disease "cluster" associated with HLA-B8
and HLA-Dw3 (Table I) can be considered autoimmune in nature in the sense
that they are associated with circulating organ or tissue specific antibodies
which are presumed to play an important, if not primary, role in the pathogenesis of the disease. The one disease category that is not autoimmune
in the sense that autoantibodies are not felt to be important in the
disease process, is gluten-sensitive enteropathy/dermatitis herpetiformis.
However, in this instance, gluten protein might be thought of as a self-
modifying antigen which leads to disease by inducing immune effector
cells which have specificity for gluten-modified self.

Systemic Lupus Erythematosus (SLE). SLE is the prototype autoimmune
disease and is characterized by the presence of circulating autoantibodies,
particularly antinuclear antibodies, as well as the deposition of immune
complexes in the vasculature and in the kidney leading to vasculitis and
nephritis. Because of the vascular abnormalities, it is a multi-system
disease with major pathologic effects manifest in the heart, brain and

TABLE I - Diseases Associated with an
Increase Frequency of HLA-B8/DRw3

	Relative Risk	
	B8	Dw3/DRw3
Gluten-sensitive Enteropathy (coeliac disease)	8.6	10.8/21.1
Dermatitis Herpetiformis	8.7	13.5/56.4
Chronic Hepatitis	8.98	/13.9
Addison's Disease	3.9	8.8/
Sicca Syndrome	3.2	19.0/
Grave's Disease (caucasians)	2.3	4.4/
Insulin-dependent Diabetes Mellitus	2.4	3.8/ 5.7
Systemic Lupus Erythematosus	2.1	/ 3.0
Sarcoidosis Arthritis	13.5	
Idiopathic Thrombocytopenic Purpura	2.9	
Tuberculosis	5.1	
Recurrent Herpes Labialis	2.5	

skin.

A great number of patients with SLE have been HLA-typed (in excess of 500) to determine the presence or absence of abnormalities in HLA antigen frequency. Initially it was found that the frequency of HLA-B8 is abnormal in that this antigen is present in almost twice the percentage of patients as in normal individuals. This gives rise to a relative risk of 1.8 to 2.1, i.e., individuals with HLA-B8 are 1.8 to 2.1 times more likely to have SLE than individuals without HLA-B8[4,5]. In some studies, the abnormality in HLA-B8 frequency was accompanied by an increase in frequency of other HLA-B locus antigens such as B5, Bw15 and Bw35, but these increases were marginal at best.

The relatively weak associations with the HLA-B8 antigen foreshadowed a more clear-cut association with HLA-D- or DR- locus antigens*[6,7]. When the frequency of various alleles in the latter locus were determined, it was found that there was an increased frequency of both HLA-Dw2 and HLA-Dw3 (in both cases present in about one half of the patients vs. about one quarter of controls). In addition it was found that about three quarters of the patients were HLA-DRw2 and DRw3 positive as contrasted with controls who were positive only one quarter of the time (relative risk in the 3-4 range).

An even stronger association between SLE and HLA antigens was found by Rienertsen et. al. using anti-B cell antisera obtained from relatively inbred multiparous women; such antisera frequently recognize B cell (and macrophage) surface antigens which are distinct from DR antigens, but which are also controlled by genes in the major histocompatibility locus. B cells of 75% of patients with SLE are positive for a particular B cell

---

*D locus antigens are identified by homozygous typing cells in mixed lymphocyte reactions; DR locus antigens are identified by antisera originally defined on homozygous typing cells; the two kinds of specificities are similar but not necessarily identical.

antigen, Ia-715, whereas only 15% of controls are positive for this antigen, leading to a relative risk of 18.8. Ia-715 is distinct from HLA-Dw2 and -Dw3 but tends to occur along with HLA-DRw1, -DRw2 and -DRw6 in the normal population. Other anti-B cell antigens (for instance, Ia-35 and Ia-172) are also found more frequently on cells obtained from SLE patients, and these antigens correlate in the normal population with HLA-DRw3.

Sicca Syndrome. Sicca syndrome (Sjogren's syndrome) is a disease characterized by lymphocytic infiltration of the exocrine glands particularly the lacrimal and salivary glands, leading to xerostomia and xerophthalmia. Infiltration of other organs results in some patients in pneumonitis, nephritis and myositis. Sicca syndrome exhibits female predominance and is associated with autoantibodies such as antinuclear antibodies and rheumatoid factor. The syndrome exists as a primary disorder with exocrine gland and/or extraglandular involvement or as a secondary disorder in which it is a feature of another disease such as rheumatoid arthritis or systemic lupus erythematosus.

In early studies HLA-B8 was found to be moderately increased in patients with sicca syndrome although not in those sicca syndrome patients with arthritis[8]. In later studies, HLA-Dw3 was found to have an even greater association with the syndrome than HLA-B8: HLA-Dw3 was present in about 80% of patients versus about 25% of controls; again the association was with those sicca patients who did not have rheumatoid arthritis[9]. An even more striking HLA association in sicca syndrome is with the B cell antigens Ia-172 and Ia-AGS; these specificities were present in all sicca patients versus 37 and 24% of controls respectively[9,10]. Ia-172 and Ia-AGS are not identical and also differ from HLA-DRw3; however they tend to occur together with HLA-DRw3,5, and 6 in normal populations.

The only HLA abnormality found in secondary sicca syndrome is an elevation in the frequency of HLA-DRw4. Thus, one may conclude that primary and secondary sicca syndrome differ on a genetic basis, with HLA-DRw3 increased in primary and HLA-DRW4 increased in secondary sicca syndrome. However, the two forms are also genetically similar in that they share one or more genes in the HLA locus that code for B cell antigens.

Endocrine Disease. The next disease or, rather, set of diseases to be considered are the endocrinopathies, Grave's disease (thyrotoxicosis), idiopathic Addison's disease, and juvenile diabetes mellitus. These diseases are clinically related in that each is associated with glandular lymphoid cell infiltration as well as organ specific antibodies. Indeed, a common etiology is suggested by the fact that they can occur together in the same individual.

Grave's Disease. As far as Grave's disease is concerned, HLA-B8 is mildly increased (relative risk 2-3) whereas HLA-Dw3 and HLA-DRw3 are moderately increased (about 50% of patients are positive for these antigens versus about 20% of controls; relative risk: 5 to 6)[11,12]. There is no increase in DRw3-positive homozygotes among patients so that the HLA gene involved is presumed to be dominant[12]. In several studies, it was found that HLA-DRw3 positive patients are less likely to remain free of thyroid disease following antithyroid drug therapy[13]. In addition, in one study HLA-B8 was associated with those patients demonstrating persistence of thyroid microsomal antibodies following withdrawal of therapy[14]. These facts suggest that HLA-B8 and HLA-DRw3 are particularly associated with these forms of thyroid disease which have immunologic factors as their basis.

In oriental (Japanese) populations wherein HLA-B8 is rare, Grave's disease is associated with HLA-Bw35[15]. This finding is of some interest since HLA-Bw35 is strongly associated (relative risk: 17) in caucasians with subacute thyroiditis, a disease characterized by subacute inflammation of the thyroid gland and fever, but unassociated with either hyperthyroidism or autoimmune phenomena.

Addison's Disease. The occurrence of HLA abnormalities with Addison's disease is not fully substantiated: HLA-B8 and HLA-Dw3 are found to be significantly increased in one report (relative risk 7 and 10-11 respectively) but in another study these antigens occurred at a normal frequency.

Diabetes Mellitus. Diabetes mellitus has been the subject of intensive study with regard to HLA abnormalities and indeed many such abnormalities have come to light[16]. Starting with the HLA-A,B, and C locus antigens, the basic facts are that juvenile, but not maturity-onset diabetes (insulin dependent, but not insulin-resistant diabetes) is associated with mild but definite increases in the prevalence of HLA-B8 as well as HLA-Bw15 and HLA-Cw3 (all in the relative risk range of 2-3); additionally, B18 rather than Bw15 is increased in French populations and HLA-Bw54 and Cw4 (rather than the antigens listed above) is increased in Japanese populations; this latter point is significant because the HLA alternate antigen to HLA-B8 in Graves disease is Bw35 not Bw54 (see discussion above). Of great importance is the fact that while the relative risk for any of the B locus antigens are only modestly increased, even in the presence of homozygosity, a sizable relative risk (9-10) obtains in those individuals with both relevant B locus antigens, B8 and Bw15. This provides the main basis for the contention that two distinct HLA genes are involved in the pathogenesis of juvenile diabetes mellitus.

The D locus antigen frequency in juvenile diabetes mellitus provides a corresponding story[16,17]. HLA-Dw3 (as well as HLA-DRw3) and HLA-Dw4 are increased to an even greater extent than the B locus antigens (relative risk in the 3-5 range). These D locus antigens are in linkage disequilibrium with HLA-B8 and HLA-Bw15 respectively and statistical analysis indicates that the B locus associations are secondary to these linkage relationships. Again relative risk in individuals with both B locus antigens is far greater than with either antigen alone.

While certain HLA B and D locus antigens are increased in juvenile diabetes mellitus, others are decreased[16,18]. Thus, in all studies HLA-B7 as well as HLA-Dw2 are present in decreased frequency in such patients; in addition, in the case of HLA-B7, a family segregation analysis was done and HLA-B7 was found to be negatively associated with diabetes[18]. This negative association is of some importance since a similar set of circumstances is found in gluten-sensitive enteropathy, as will be discussed at some length below.

Family studies which focus on families containing several siblings with juvenile diabetes mellitus have been performed by several groups[19,21]. In all of these studies, it was found that the vast majority of affected siblings share at least one HLA haplotype and at least half share both HLA haplotypes. One set of authors, whose data show that greater than 90% of affected siblings were HLA-identical, concluded that juvenile diabetes was due to a single recessive gene[21]. These authors attribute the small percentage of nonidentical siblings to either HLA locus recombinations (which they claim were higher in diabetic families than in normal families) or to homozygosity for the putative diabetes disease gene in a parent (although none of the parents were diabetic). Other authors, whose data show that 30-50% of affected siblings are not HLA identical, have concluded that juvenile diabetes millitus is due to two dominant but separate genes which are more likely to occur together in the HLA identical siblings but can occur together in the nonidentical sibs as well[20]. This view must be considered the most likely one, especially in light of the additive relative risk obtained when two separate B locus antigens are present. In addition, evidence is now appearing that diabetes mellitus patients bearing B8-DRw3 alone or Bw15-DRw4 alone may differ immunologically. The relevant data here is that B8-DRW3 bearing patients are more likely to have persistance of anti-B cell antibodies and have associated autoimmune diseases whereas Bwl5-DRw4 patients are more likely to have high titers of antibodies to exogenous insulin[22,23]. These immunologic data again suggest that diabetes mellitus is associated with the presence of two distinct HLA genes.

<u>Myasthenia Gravis</u>. Myasthenia gravis is another disease in which a clearcut association with HLA-B8 and HLA-Dw3 has been shown. This disease is an abnormality of neuromuscular function which results in muscle weakness. Its pathogenesis is related to neuromuscular blockade due, at least in some cases, to an autoantibody that has specificity for the acetylcholine receptor. One group of patients consists of those with thymic hyperplasia associated with intrathymic germinal centers; these patients usually have early onset disease. Another group of patients consist of those with thymomas; this group usually consists of patients with late onset disease. Finally, in common with many of the other autoimmune diseases discussed above, the disease shows female predominance.

HLA-B8 has been repeatedly found to be increased in myasthenia gravis with a relative risk in the 4-5 range for the total patient group[24]. However, a considerably more impressive association with HLA-B8 is found if only myasthenia gravis patients with early onset disease and/or patients with thymic hyperplasia are considered: these patients have a 50-60% frequency of HLA-B8 (relative risk greater than 5)[24,25]. The other side of the coin is that HLA-B8 is not increased in patients with thymoma and for patients with late onset disease.

HLA-Dw3 and DRw3 also show an increase in a same subset of patients who are characterized by a HLA-B8 increase[25,26]. However, in contrast to the previously discussed HLA-B8-associated diseases, the HLA-Dw3 association is less impressive than the HLA-B8 association, suggesting that in this case the "disease gene" is in closer linkage disequilibrium with the B locus gene than the D locus gene[26].

Chronic Active Hepatitis. Chronic active hepatitis is yet another disease associated with HLA-B8. As indicated by Mackay, this association depends on the delineation of a more or less homogeneous subset of patients with "autoimmune" chronic hepatitis which is defined by early onset, female predominance, certain extra-hepatic features, presence of smooth muscle antibody and/or anti-nuclear antibody and very high gamma globulin levels[27]. This classification would specifically exclude disease associated with the presence of hepatitis B viral antigen, HB_sAg, as well as drug-associated hepatitis and chronic hepatitis unassociated with autoantibodies or Hb_sAg.

HLA-B8 has been shown to be significantly increased in numerous studies of autoimmune chronic active hepatitis: 60-70% of patients are HLA-B8 positive versus about 20% of control patients (relative risk about 3). A similar increase in HLA-Dw3 has been reported, yielding a similar relative risk for this antigen[28]; hence, in this case, the disease gene seems equally associated with the B locus and D locus antigens. As in other B8/Dw3 associations, the HLA-B8-negative group of CAH patients have fewer autoimmune reactions and were more easily treated. Finally, HLA-B8 is not consistently increased in other forms of chronic hepatitis or in alcoholic cirrhosis.

Gluten-Sensitive Enteropathy. The last association with HLA-B8 and HLA-Dw3 to be discussed is the one with gluten-sensitive enteropathy (GSE) (coeliac sprue disease) and dermatitis herpetiformis, disease entities where the association is strongest and the relative risk is highest[29]. In both of these conditions, patients demonstrate intestinal villous atrophy and malabsorption which is due to gluten-protein toxicity. The nature of the mechanism through which gluten affects this change is unclear, but there is ample evidence that patients respond to gluten immunologically and it seems likely that the intestinal injury is mediated by an immunologic process. In dermatitis herpetiformis (DH), a gastrointestinal (GI) abnormality entirely similar to that found in gluten-sensitive enteropathy occurs, but in this case the GI lesion is associated with a vesicular skin lesion characterized by subepithelial IgA deposits.

HLA-B8 is found in 70 to 80% of GSE patients (relative risk 8 to 9) originating from northern Europe and the United States[29]. The prevalence of this antigen among patients in southern Germany and Austria is somewhat lower, about 60%, but still significantly greater than the prevalence in normal individuals[30]. As might be expected, the frequency of HLA-B8 in well diagnosed dermatitis herpetiformis patients is even higher than that in GSE patients; in this case the prevalence is in the 90% range.[31]

Another B locus antigen abnormality in GSE is the somewhat decreased incidence of HLA-B7; in this respect GSE is similar to juvenile diabetes mellitus. Additionally, HLA-A1 is increased in GSE, but this the result of linkage disequilibrium. In family studies, it was shown that GSE segregates with HLA-B8, but HLA identical siblings are frequently observed who are disease free, suggesting the presence of other environmental or genetic factors. The former is strengthened by the knowledge that several sets of discordant identical twins have been observed. Finally, it should also be mentioned that in families with more than one affected sibling, the siblings with disease are never completely HLA-nonidentical. This indicates that an HLA gene is necessary, if not sufficient, for disease.

HLA-Dw3 and DRw3 is also increased in GSE[32] and, in fact, this antigen is present at a greater frequency than HLA-B8: an 80-95% prevalence rate is found giving a relative risk of greater than 70. Analysis of the B8 and Dw3 associations discloses that the HLA-Dw3 occurred in patients whether or not HLA-B8 was present whereas HLA-B8 occurred only when Dw3 was present. Thus, the GSE "disease gene" appears to be more closely linked to the D locus than the B locus HLA antigen, in common with many, but not all, of the diseases mentioned above.

Recently another D locus antigen has found to be increased in patients with GSE, HLA-DRw7[33]. However, this increase is found only in patients located in certain geographical areas, namely, Spain and Italy (not in Holland or the United States). In the one study reported, this increase accompanied the HLA-DRw3 increase and the relative risk of individuals with both antigens was increased over those with either one alone. Thus, in selected populations, it is possible that two disease genes, each in linkage disequilibrium with a separate D locus gene may be present.

Additional cell surface markers particularly associated with GSE have been sought using antiserums obtained from mothers of GSE patients. In this novel approach, the underlying concept is that mothers may be immunized during pregnancy with antigens present on cells present in the fetus. In fact, several maternal antiserums have been identified which do react with patient (GSE and DH) B cells in a high percentage of cases (70-90%) but only a low (but definite) percentage of cells from normal individuals[34]. The specificities identified in this way are discordant with D locus specificities in that the identifying antiserums do not react with defined homozygous D locus cells, including cells bearing HLA-Dw3. Thus, these maternal antiserums are identifying antigens which are distinct from known D locus specificities. Finally, a family study has been reported in which members were typed for HLA-B and D locus as well as for the GSE-associated B cell antigen described above which is identified with the maternal antiserums[35]. In several instances, HLA B and D locus nonidentical sibs were identified who were nevertheless positive for GSE-associated B cell antigens. This and related findings suggest that in contrast to the B cell antigens which are increased in SLE and sicca syndrome, the GSE-associated B cell antigen is controlled by a non-HLA gene. Thus, the picture that is emerging in GSE is that this disease is a multigenic defect associated with one or more HLA genes as well as at least one non-HLA gene. Furthermore, inheritance of the disease depends on the simultaneous presence of the several genes involved. This view has received support from a mathematical analysis of the genetics of GSE which allows prediction of the incidence of this disease in both populations and families[36].

Individual Diseases Associated with HLA Abnormalities Other than HLA-B8 and HLA-Dw3. The HLA-B8/DW3 antigens are by no means the only HLA antigens associated with disease, or even autoimmune disease. In the section below the most important of these associations are discussed; in addition, in Table II are listed a series of other diseases in which significant HLA-disease associations have been found.

Multiple Sclerosis (MS). Multiple sclerosis is an inflammatory disease of the central nervous system characterized by discrete areas of demyelinization (plaques) in the white matter which result in disturbed impulse propagation. The disease may be due to viral infection, a subtle

Table II Miscellaneous HLA Associations with Disease

	HLA Antigen	Relative Risk
Behcet's Disease	B5	4 - 6
Takayasu's Disease (Japanese)	B5 Bw52	4 5 - 6
IgA Mesangial glomerulo nephritis	Bw35	4 - 5
Cryptogenic fibrosing alveolitis	B12	9 - 10
Buerger's disease	A9	6 - 7
Idiopathic hemachromatosis	A3 B14	8 - 9 9 - 10
de Quervain's thyroiditis	Bw35	16 - 17
Pemphigus Vulgaris (Jews)	A10	5 - 6

disturbance in immune function, or both.

Initially, a weak association between HLA-B7 (as well as HLA-A3 which is in linkage disequilibrium with HLA-B7) was found with a relative risk in the 1.8-2.5 range[36]; in addition, HLA-Bw12 was found to be decreased, probably as a compensatory phenomenon. More recently, a far stronger association between MS and HLA-Dw2/DRw2 has been established[36]. These latter antigens are found in about 50-70% of the patients versus about 20% of normals, giving a relative risk of 4 or more. In addition, DRw3 is also increased and over 75% of patients have either DRw2 or DRw3 compared to about 40% of controls. The increase in DRw3 explains a previous finding of consistent but statistical insignificant increases in HLA-B8.

Paty et. al. found that immune responses to herpes simplex virus (lymphocyte proliferation) but not herpes zoster virus was significantly decreased in MS patients bearing HLA-Dw2 but not those patients not bearing this antigen[37]. This suggests the HLA-Dw2 may be in linkage disequilibrium with an immune suppressor gene which is specific for certain antigens. As a result, patients with MS may be unable to respond to certain viral antigens and viral infections are then established which cause disease.

Goodpasture's Syndrome. Goodpasture's syndrome, a disease characterized by nephritis, lung hemorrhage and antiglomerular basement membrane antibodies, has an even stronger association with HLA-DRw2 than does MS[38]. In this disease, fully 88% of patients are DRw2-positive versus 32% of normal individuals (relative risk 15.9). Additionally, HLA-A3 and HLA-B7 are modestly increased. Since relapse in Goodpasture's syndrome is precipitated by infection, here, as in patients with MS there is the suggestion that an environmental agent, perhaps a virus, is a causative agent.

Adult and Juvenile Rheumatoid Arthritis. Another important group of HLA-B and D locus associations is that between HLA antigens and various arthropathies. In adult rheumatoid arthritis, while A locus and B locus antigen frequencies are normal, a D locus antigen association is quite definitely present: HLA-Dw4 is present in 70% of patients versus 28% of controls (relative risk 6.0)[39]. Again, in juvenile rheumatoid arthritis, A and B locus antigens are present in normal frequency whereas two D locus antigens, HLA-Dw7 and HLA-Dw8 are increased[40]. In addition, another D locus antigen defined by homozygous cells obtained from a juvenile rheumatoid arthritis patient and termed TMo was also significantly associated with this form of arthritis, particularly a clinical form known as persistent pauci-articular rheumatoid arthritis (relative risk 67.7)[40].

Psoriasis and Psoriatic Arthritis. Finally, significant HLA abnormalities have been found in patients with psoriasis, both those with and without psoriatic arthritis. HLA-B13, HLA-B17 and HLA-Cw6, the latter a C locus antigen, are increased in frequency in both patient groups[41,42]. Additionally, in patients with psoriatic arthritis, HLA-A26, HLA-B27 and HLA-B38 are elevated as well[41]. As far as D locus antigens are concerned, DRw7 is elevated in patients with and without arthritis whereas DRw4 is elevated only in patients with arthritis[43]. From this complex picture, it is apparent that while psoriasis and psoriatic arthritis are similar in that they share common skin manifestations, they are different in that they are associated with different HLA patterns.

The multiplicity of associations in both forms of psoriasis raises the possibility that more than one gene in the major histocompatibility complex is necessary for disease expression. This possibility is also suggested by the fact that the antigen doublet HLA-Cw6 and HLA-DRw7 appear together more frequently in patients than in normals, whereas the antigen triplet HLA-Cw6, HLA-B17 and HLA-DRw7 is not increased in frequency; since the HLA-Cw6 and the HLA-DRw7 genes map on either side of HLA-B17, these genes are not likely to be occurring in psoriasis together because of linkage disequilibrium, but rather because each is associated with a separate gene necessary for the disease[43].

Possible Mechanisms Underlying an Association of HLA-B8/Dw3 and Disease.
Having documented the association of two relatively common HLA types,
HLA-B8 and HLA-Dw3 (DRw3) with a variety of diseases, we must now turn
our attention to the possible mechanisms which could account for this
association. In this regard, the overriding fact is that the diseases in
question are autoimmune diseases and one must therefore consider the
possibility that the HLA antigens associated with these diseases play a key
role in the production of the autoimmunity. This possibility may take one
or both of two forms: on the one hand the HLA genes in question (HLA-B8/Dw3)
or genes in linkage disequilibrium with these genes may somehow code for a
general, more or less nonspecific abnormality of immune responsiveness; as
such the genes responsible for this general abnormality may ordinarily
provide a selective advantage to those individuals who bear them and may
lead to disease only when they are present in conjunction with other
genetic and/or environmental factors; on the other hand, the HLA genes in
question may be associated with autoimmune states because they are in
linkage disequilibrium with specific and unique genes which cause immunologic
abnormalities affecting certain specific immune responses rather than
immune responses generally. A third possibility is a composite of the
first two, namely that the genes coding for HLA-B8/Dw3 or genes in linkage
disequilibrium with these genes, cause disease through a general abnormality
of immune responsiveness but only in the presence of other genes which
code for complementary and specific abnormalities of the immune response.

The evidence supporting the first concept, i.e., that the genes coding
for HLA-B8/Dw3 (or linked genes) are responsible for a general and nonspecific
abnormality shared by all autoimmune diseases is basically of two types:
1) evidence derived from studies which support the notion that normal
individuals bearing HLA-B8 and/or HLA-Dw3 (HLA-B8/Dw3) hyper-respond to

various immunologic stimuli; and 2) studies of autoimmune states per se which indicate that individuals with autoimmunity have a general defect in the regulation of specific and/or nonspecific immune responses, wherein they fail to limit or suppress immune responses.

Perhaps the best evidence for altered responsiveness in normal individuals bearing HLA-B8 is derived from the work of Osoba and Falk[44]. These investigators studied mixed lymphocyte responses in a large number of normal individuals using a constant panel of cryopreserved stimulator cells. They then correlated the magnitude of the response (quantitated by thymidine incorportion) with HLA type. Of great interest was the fact that only one A or B locus HLA type (no D locus correlations were made) had a statistically significant greater response than that observed for the entire group: individuals with HLA-B8. It should be noted that the excess of HLA-B-positive individuals among the hyper-responders was not very marked, yet this excess would make the difference between health and disease in a variety of situations, particularly if allowance is made for possible amplification effects within the immune system.

Several other studies indicating an occurrence of abnormal responsiveness in normal individuals bearing HLA-B8 are extant: 1) Galbraith et. al. have shown that antibody titres to a variety of viral and tissue antigens were significantly greater in HLA-B8 positive than in HLA-B8 negative patients with HB_sAg-negative chronic active hepatitis[45]; similarly, Scott et. al. have shown that anti-gluten protein antibody levels in patients with liver disease who were HLA-B8 positive were higher than those with liver disease who were HLA-B8 negative[46]. In both of these studies it is possible that the liver disease present unveiled the latent ability of individuals to respond or not to respond to environmental antigens; 2) Cunningham-Rundles et. al. have shown that in vitro proliferative responses of normal cells to gluten-protein was greater if the cells were obtained from normal HLA-B8 positive individuals rather than normal HLA-B8 negative individuals; in contrast, no difference in these two groups' capacity to respond to candida antigen was seen[47]; 3) finally, Bach and his colleagues have shown that HLA-B8 positive individuals on renal dialysis therapy had a greater capacity to clear HB_sAg antigen than HLA-B8 negative individuals[48].

Obviously these studies in normal individuals are not yet sufficient to substantiate the idea that HLA-B8/HLA-Dw3 is associated with immunologic hyper-responsiveness. Additional studies with other antigens and other kinds of immune responses must be done. In this regard, there have been a number of studies of the relationship between magnitude of the response to specific viral antigens and HLA type. In these studies, specific HLA associations have indeed been observed, but no single HLA antigen, let alone HLA-B8/Dw3, has been found to be associated with hyper-responsiveness. For instance, HLA-DHO is associated in Japanese populations with decreased antitetanus toxoid responses[49], HLA-Bwl6 is associated with decreased anti-live influenza A responses (but normal responses to killed organisms)[50], and HLA-Cw3 and HLA-Bw40 is associated with decreased responses to vaccinia[51]. These associations may be due to the presence of specific immune response or suppressor genes in linkage disequilibrium with the HLA genes in question, a possibility suggested above for HLA associations with disease states. In any case, the lack of association between HLA-B8/Dw3 with these various responses to viral antigens leads to the suggestion that hyper-responsiveness associated with HLA-B8/Dw3 does not apply to all immune responses and may in fact be limited to certain classes of antigens.

Turning now to the evidence for hyper-responsiveness derived from the study of the autoimmune disease states, we find that in several instances autoimmune diseases have been associated with decreases in the number or activity of suppressor T-cells. In representative studies supporting this observation, peripheral blood cells obtained from patients with autoimmunity such as those with systemic lupus erythematosus are stimulated with a T cell mitogen, conconavalin A (Con A) a substance known to stimulate suppressor cell activity[52]. The stimulated cells are then washed and added to an indicator system consisting of peripheral blood lymphoid cells being stimulated by a mitogen to undergo proliferation and/or Ig synthesis. Con A-stimulated cells obtained from normal individuals inhibits such proliferation and/or Ig synthesis whereas Con A stimulated cells obtained from patients have a greatly reduced capacity to inhibit such proliferation and/or synthesis. In the sense that patients with SLE manifest decreased suppressor T cell function and persistent immunoglobulin synthesis in situations where normal individuals show suppressed responses, such patients can be said to be nonspecifically hyper-responsive.

Other autoimmune states associated with HLA-B8/DRw3 where similar defects in non-specific suppressor T cell function has been found is myasthenia gravis and chronic hepatitis[53,54]. However, no evidence for such an abnormality has been found in sicca syndrome, although it can hardly be said that this disease state has been exhaustively studied[55]. Additionally, deficient suppressor T cell abnormalities have been described in at least one disease wherein HLA-B8/DRw3 is clearly not increased, primary biliary cirrhosis. One must therefore come to the conclusion that even if the gene controlling HLA-B8/DRw3 is linked to a gene controlling immune regulation in a variety of diseases, the latter gene can occur in the absence of immunoregulatory abnormalities and vice versa.

Proceeding now to a consideration of the possible mechanism that might underlie the relationship between an HLA gene and immunoregulation, one may draw on the recently obtained evidence that at least two autoimmune diseases, SLE and primary biliary cirrhosis, are marked by defective autologous mixed lymphocyte reactions, and there is some cause to believe that such reactions might be critical to the maintenance of normal regulatory T cell function[56,57]. To understand this line of reasoning we must first be aware of certain facts: 1) the autologous mixed lymphocyte reaction (autologous MLR) is a proliferative response of purified T cells upon exposure to purified autologous non-T cells; 2) whereas neither the precise cell type within the non-T cell population responsible for stimulation nor the precise antigen on the non-T cell surface involved in stimulation is known, the stimulating antigen is likely to be coded for by a HLA gene; and finally 3) in recent studies, it has been shown that cells stimulated in the autologous MLR are at least partially distinct from those stimulated in the allogeneic MLR; in addition, the suppressor T cell induced by Con A is among the T cell population stimulated in the autologuos MLR rather than in the T cell population stimulated by the allogeneic MLR. These facts, taken together, lead to the possibility that an autologous MLR occurring under physiological circumstances is necessary for suppressor T cell development. It is but a short step from this thesis to the concept that a gene in the HLA region in linkage disequilibrium with HLA-Dw3/DRw3 can somehow control autologous MLR responses and thereby suppressor T cell function.

So far in our discussion of the association of HLA with a variety of autoimmune diseases, we have been focusing on the possibility that a common gene is present which is responsible for the nonspecific abnormality. As indicated above, however, it is also important to consider the possibility that the HLA genes in question are, in each of the disease states, in linkage disequilibrium with a unique disease gene. Furthermore, the possibility must be considered that the disease genes are, in reality, immune response genes (Ir genes) or immune suppressor (Is genes which allow responses (or cause lack of responses) to specific antigens which are uniquely important to the pathogenesis of each of the disease states under consideration. Within this context, these Ir disease genes can act in

either of two ways: 1) the genes can code for "structural" determinants
which dictate the selection of one or more lymphoid clones that are capable
of reacting with unmodified cell surface antigens/self antigens); normally
such clones are deleted during the process of clonal selection during
ontogeny whereas the clones that react only with modified cell determinants
are allowed to survive; 2) the genes can code for regulatory processes
which act in a specific way on the control of the level of response to
particular antigens; in this view the regulatory T cells (suppressor T
cells and helper T cells) dedicated to the control of responses to specific
antigens are somehow in a configuration that causes hyper-responsiveness
to particular autoantigens.

No direct evidence in favor of the existence of unique disease genes
of these sorts is extant. However, as mentioned above in the discussion of
the individual diseases associated with HLA-B8/Dw3 abnormalities, certain
more specific B cell antigens have been found in increased frequency in
such diseases as SLE and sicca syndrome (e.g., Ia 175, Ia-Ags). Thus, it
is at least theoretically possible that the genes controlling these antigens
are in fact the specific immune response genes which act in the manner
described above. Another possibility, one more compatible with the fact
that the B cell antigens do occur in normal individuals, is that the cell
surface molecules important to the induction and regulation of immune
responses are comprised of amino acid sequences controlled by two or more
HLA-locus genes; on this basis it is possible that certain combinations of
non-unique HLA genes can give rise to unique cell surface molecules which
then lead to specific immune responses as well as specific diseases.

A phenomenon which will require explanation if the view that HLA
associations with disease can be accounted for by postulating that disease
genes (specific or nonspecific) are in linkage disequilibrium with HLA-B8/Dw3
genes is the fact that for some reason there are a limited set of HLA

genes, for instance those controlling HLA-B8/Dw3, that is in linkage

disequilibrium with a variety of disease genes. A possible explanation of

this fact is that HLA-B8 and HLA-Dw3 is in linkage to disequilibrium with

disease genes because these antigens are not mere marker genes and do in

fact provide some necessary element in the development of the disease

process. In support of this possibility, one might mention first that HLA

antigens coded for by A,B and D locus genes are cell surface molecules

which participate in cell-cell interactions important to the immune response.

For instance, cytotoxic T cells recognize antigens only if the antigen is

directly modifying HLA antigen (modified self recognition) or is at least

closely associated with HLA antigen (dual recognition). Similarly, macrophage

presentation of antigen to T cell involves both the antigen and HLA gene

products (Ia antigen). In view of these facts, the possibility comes into

view that cells bearing HLA-B8/DRw3 give rise to particularly immunogenic

signals or result in particularly "vulnerable" targets when modified by or

associated with certain kinds of antigens. This could occur for two

reasons, on the one hand, certain HLA antigens, because of intrinsic

structural features, more readily result in the clonal selection of lymphoid

clones capable of reacting with antigen modifying or associated with those

HLA-antigens; on the other hand, certain HLA genes may be linked to regu-

latory genes which provide for increased responses to antigens modifying or

associated with the HLA antigens coded by those HLA genes; in this way,

sets of HLA genes work in tandem to result in greater or lesser immune

responses.

This latter idea could form the basis of the selective advantage thought

to underlie the phenomenon of linkage disequilibrium in that certain A,B and

D locus genes could be linked to other HLA genes which result in a strong

response for antigens associated with the A,B and D locus alleles coded for

by the former set of genes. In this way an individual with a given set of

HLA alleles would have a selective advantage for a given immune function because he would automatically inherit a high capacity to respond to antigens associated on the cell surface with his HLA antigens. It is obvious that this selective advantage, however, could have a negative side. The individual with certain sets of HLA genes could, in the presence of yet other genetic and environmental factors also have a tendency to hyper-respond to modified self-antigens and autoimmunity may result.

These possibilities receives some support from the recent work of Shaw and Biddison[59,60]. These authors induced cytotoxic effector T cells specific for influenza virus by adding this virus to cultured cells. As in murine systems, they found that the effector cells killed influenza virus-modified target cells in direct relation to the extent with which they shared HLA antigens with the effector cell. More to the point, they showed, in family studies, that certain individuals preferentially lysed target cells bearing the maternal haplotype whereas other preferentially lysed target cells bearing the paternal haplotype. Related differencies in patterns of lysis was also seen in unrelated individuals: cells from individuals who share HLA type may nevertheless differ in their ability to lyse virus-modified target cells bearing similar HLA antigens. These results suggest that an HLA gene determines the magnitude of reponse to virus-modified HLA gene products either by acting as a structural gene capable of inducing a strong immune response or as a result of association with regulatory genes which provide for a high level of response to certain antigens associated on the cell surface with the HLA antigen, coded for by the HLA gene. In terms of the present discussion, it is possible that cells bearing HLA-B8/Dw3 when modified by certain antigens induce particularly vigorous responses to these antigens either because the genes controlling HLA-B8/Dw3 also lead to large responses or because the genes controlling HLA-B8/Dw3 are linked to regulatory genes which provide for high responses to certain antigens associated with HLA-B8/Dw3.

Possible mechanisms underlying the association of various B and D locus antigens other than HLA-B8/DW3 with disease. The possible mechanisms operative in the association of various HLA antigens other than HLA-B8/Dw3 suchas that of HLA-B7/Dw2 with multiple sclerosis and HLA-Dw4 with rheumatoid arthritis is best discussed within the context of the HLA-B8/Dw3 association. In this regard, the same general principles are likely operative for HLA-B8/Dw3 are likely to hold:

1) The mechanisms probably involve subtle alteration in immunologic responses since the diseases involved are widely regarded as involving immunologic dysfunction; 2) the actual disease genes are not those coding for the HLA antigens per se but rather are in linkage disequilibrium with such HLA genes; 3) the actual disease genes may involve antigen-specific events in which case they would be equivalent to classical immune response genes which are described in inbred rodents and guinea pigs; 4) the actual disease genes may involve antigen non-specific events, in which case they would control general responsiveness or responsiveness to certain classes of antigens; here the possibility must be considered that the abnormality of responsiveness may involve hypo-responsiveness as well as hyper-responsiveness, as for example, decreased responses to certain classes of viral antigens leading to chronic infection with the viruses; and 5) the genes controlling HLA antigens may sometimes play a more active role in the disease process; i.e., may be more than simple marker genes. In this regard, the HLA genes may act in tandem with linked regulatory genes to produce a given abnormality.

An additional possibility not considered previously, is that the HLA gene product may provide a binding site for products of disease producing organisms or other toxic materials. The best evidence that this mechanism may occur is inherent in the recent work of Geczy et. al.[61]. These workers have shown that antisera produced in response to immunization with certain klebsiellia stains react with lymphocytes obtained from HLA-B27 positive patients with ankylosing spondylitis (AS) but not with lymphocytes of HLA-B27 negative ankylosing spondylitis patients. Furthermore, a factor or factors in klebsiella culture can modify HLA-B27 positive cells from AS negative individuals so that they too react with the anti-klebsiella antisera. The results suggest that a klebsiella antigen can modify or bind to B27 positive lymphocytes and that this may be a critical step in the production of ankylosing spondylitis.

For completeness, one might mention several additional mechanisms through which HLA antigens are associated with disease. In this regard, there is the "molecular mimicry" argument in which HLA antigens are assumed to be similar or identical to antigens in the environment which are capable of inciting a pathologic state (virus or other toxic entity). As a result the individual either cannot respond to the agent appropriately because it is regarded as self or responds appropriately to the agent as well as inappropriately to cross-reactive self-antigens. In a varient of this theme, HLA antigens are assumed to be present in the coat of a pathogenic virus as a result of viral budding and the virus subsequently evokes responses against viral antibodies as well as self-HLA antigens so as to induce autoimmunity. It should be emphasized that while these mechanisms are quite plausible, they have not been experimentally substantiated in any disease entity and should be regarded as theoretical constructs which are useful only for orienting further research.

Summary

In summary, a large fraction of the associations between HLA antigens and disease consists of the association of certain HLA antigens (particularly HLA-B8/DW3) with autoimmune states. These associations can be accounted for by the existence of one or more common immunoregulatory genes which are in linkage disequilibrium with the HLA B and D locus genes and which codes for altered responsiveness to at least certain classes of antigens. It also can be explained by the occurrence by a large number of more specific disease genes in linkage disequilibrium with the HLA-B and -D locus genes which act as abnormal immune response genes governing responses to self or modified self antigens. The reason for the associations of the genes controlling specific HLA genes with either the nonspecific or the specific disease genes is unknown. It may relate to the fact that in most instances this association provides a selective advantage and it is only the concomitance of yet other genetic or environmental factors that results in disease. A concept that is beginning to emerge from the facts surrounding HLA asociations with disease is that the associations are based on multiple gene interactions and, as a corollary to this, one does not have to postulate a single disease gene linked to HLA genes; rather, it appears that the simultaneous presence of several different HLA (and non-HLA) genes, each present in varying frequency in normal individuals, is sufficient to result in disease.

From this short review of the field it is obvious that a great deal more concerning the specifics of HLA associations with autoimmune disease needs to be delineated. In this regard it is important now that the field move beyond the discovery of simple associations between HLA and disease and move into the detailed study of the mechanism by which these associations actually lead to altered pathophysiology.

REFERENCES

1. Dausset, J. 1977. Clinical Implications (Nosology, Diagnosis, Prognosis and Preventive Therapy) in HLA and disease. J. Dausset and A. Svejgaard, Ed. Munksgaard, Copenhagen. p. 298.
2. Day, N. K., P. L'Esperance, R. A. Good, et. al. 1975. Hereditary C2 deficiency: genetic studies and association with the HLA system. J. Exp. Med. 141:1464.
3. Levine, L. S., M. Zachmann, M. I. New et. al. 1978. Genetic mapping of the 21-hydroxylase-deficiency within the HLA linkage group. N. Eng. J. Med. 299:911.

4. Grumet, F. C., A. Conkell, J. G. Bodmer, et. al. 1971. Histocompatibility (HLA-A) antigens associated with systemic lupus erythematosus: a possible genetic predisposition to disease. N. Eng. J. Med. 285:193.
5. Kissmeyer-Nielsen, F., K. E. Kjerbye, E. Andersen, et. al. 1975. HLA Antigens in systemic lupus erythematosus. Transplantation Rev. 22:164.
6. Reinertsen, J. L., J. H. Klippel, A. H. Johnson et. al. 1978. B-lymphocyte alloantigens associated with systemic lupus erythematosus. N. Eng. J. Med. 299:515.
7. Gibofsky, A., R. J. Winchester, M. Patarroyo et. al. 1978. Disease associations of the Ia-like human alloantigens contrasting patterns in rheumatoid arthritis and systemic lupus erythematosus. J. Exp. Med. 148:1728.
8. Svejgaard, A. and L. P. Ryder 1977. Associations between HLA and disease. In: HLA and Disease. J. Dausset and A. Svejgaard, Eds. Munksgaard, Copenhagen. p. 46.
9. Chused, T. M., S. S. Kassan, S. S., G., Opelz, et. al. (1977). Sjogren's syndrome associated with HLA-Dw3. N. Eng. J. Med. 296:895.
10. Moutsopoulos, A. M., T. M. Chused, A. H. Johnson et. al. 1978. B-lymphocyte alloantigens in sicca syndrome. Science 199:1441.
11. Thorsby, E. E. Segaard, J. H. Solean and L. Kornstad 1975. The frequency of major histocompatibility antigens (SD & LD) in thyrotoxicosis. Tissue Antigens 6:54.
12. Farid, N. R., L. Sampson, E. P. Noel, et. al. 1979. The study of human leucocyte D locus related antigens in Grave's disease. J. Clin. Invest. 63:108.
13. Bech, K., B. Lumhotz, J. Nerup et. al. 1977. HLA antigens in Grave's disease. Acta Endocrinol. 86:510.
14. Irvine, W. J., R. S. Gray, P. J. Morris et. al. 1977. Correlation of HLA and antithyroid antibodies with clinical course of thyrotoxicosis treated with other thyroid drugs. Lancet II: 898.
15. Nerup, J., Cr. Cathelineau, J. Seignalet et. al. 1977. HLA and endocrine diseases. In: HLA and Disease. J. Dausset and A. Svejgaard, Eds. Menksgaard, Copenhagen. p. 149.
16. Nerup, J. 1978. HLA studies in diabetes mellitus: a review. Adv. in Metab. Disorders 9:263.
17. De Moerloose, P. H., X. Chardonnens, P. Vassali, et. al. 1977. Antigenes HLA-D de lymphocyte B et susceptibilite a certaines maladies. Schweiz. Med. Wochenshr. 107:1461.
18. Van de Patte, I., C. Vermylen, P. Decraene et. al. 1976. Segregation of HLA-B7 in juvenile-onset diabetes mellitus. Lancet II. 251.
19. Cudworth, A. G., J. C. Woodrow 1975. Evidence for HLA-linked genes in "juvenile" diabetes mellitus. Brit. Med. J. 3:133.
20. Barbosa, J. R. King, H. Noreen, et. al. 1977. The histocompatibility system in juvenile, insulin-dependent diabetes multiplex kindreds. J. Clin. Invest. 60:989.
21. Rubinstein, P., N. Suciu-Foca, J. F. Nicholson 1977. Genetics of juvenile diabetes mellitus. A recessive gene closely linked to HLA-D and with 50 per cent penetrance. N. Eng. J. Med. 297:1036.
22. Morris, P. J., H. Vaughn, W. J. Irvine et. al. 1976. HLA and pancreatic islet cell antibodies in diabetes. Lancet II:652.
23. Bertrams, J., F. K. Jansen, D. Gruneklee, et. al. 1976. HLA antigens and immuno-responsiveness to insulin in insulin-dependent diabetes mellitus. Tissue Antigens 8:13.
24. Fritz, D., C. Herrman, Jr., F. Naeim et. al. 1974. HLA-antigens in myasthenia gravis. Lancet I:240.

25. Safwenberg, J., L. Hammerstrom and J. B. Lindblom 1978. HLA-A, -B, -C, and -D antigens in male patients with myasthenia gravis. Tissue Antigens 12:136.
26. Moller, E., L. Hammerstrom and E. Smith 1976. HL-A8 and LD-8a in patients with myasthenia gravis. Tissue Antigens 7:39.
27. Mackay, I. R. 1977. HLA and Liver Disease. In: HLA and Disease. J. Dausset and A. Svejgaard, Eds. Munksgaard; Copenhagen. p. 186.
28. Opelz, G., 1977. HLA determinants in chronic active liver disease: possible relation of HLA-Dw3 to prognosis. Tissue Antigens 9:36.
29. Strober, W. 1977. Abnormalities of the HLA system and gastrointestinal disease. In: HLA and Disease. J. Dausset and A. Svejgaard, Eds. Munksgaard, Copenhagen. p. 168.
30. Harms, K., G. Granditsch, E. Rossipal, et. al. 1974. HLA in patients with coeilac disease and their families. In: Proc. 2nd Internat. Coeilac Symp. W. Th. J. M. Hekkens and A. S. Pena, Eds. Stenfert-Kroese, Leiden. p. 215.
31. Katz, S. I., K. C. Hertz, G. N. Rogentine, et. al., 1977. HLA-B8 and dermatitis herpetiformis in patients with IgA deposits in skin. Arch. of Dermatology. 113:155.
32. Keuning, J. J., A. S. Pena, A. van Leeuwen, HLA-Dw3 association with coeliac disease. Lancet I:506.
33. DeMarchi, M., I. Borelli, E. Olivetti, et. al. 1979. Two HLA-D and DR alleles are associated with coeliac disease. Tissue Antigens 14:309.
34. Mann, D. L., S. I. Katz, D. L. Nelson, et al. 1976. Specific B cell antigens associated with gluten-sensitive enteropathy and dermatitis herpetiformis. Lancet I.:110
35. Pena, A. S., D. L. Mann, N. E. Hague, et. al. 1978. The genetic basis of gluten-sensitive enteropathy. Gastroenterology 75:230.
36. Jersild, C., B. Dupont, T. Fog, et al. 1975. Histocompatibility determinants in multiple sclerosis. Trans Reviews 22:148.
37. Paty, D. W., H. K. Cousin, C. R. Stiller, et. al. 1977. HLA-D typing with an association of Dw2 and absent immune responses toward herpes simplex (type I) antigen in multiple sclerosis. Transplant. Proc. 9:1845.
38. Reese, A. J., D. K. Peters, D A .S. Compston, et al.1978. Strong association between HLA-DRw2 and antibody mediated Goodpasture's syndrome. Lancet I:966.
39. Stastny, P. 1978. Association of the B cell alloantigen DRw4 with rheumatoid arthritis. N. Eng. J. Med. 298:869.
40. Stastny, P., and C. W. Fink. 1979. Different HLA-D associations in adult and juvenile rheumatoid arthritis. J. Clin. Invest. 63:124.
41. Roux, H., P. Meruer, D. Maestracci, et. al. Psoriatic arthritis and HLA antigens 1977. J. Rheumatol. (Suppl.) 3:64.
42. McMichael, A. J., V. Morhenn, R. Payne, et. al. HLA C and D antigens associated with psoriasis. Br. J. Dermatology 98:287.
43. Mann, D. L. and C. Murray 1979. HLA alloantigens: disease association and biologic significance. Seminars in Hemat. 16:293.
44. Osoba, D. and J. Falk, 1978. HLA-B8 phenotype associated with an increased mixed leukocyte reaction. Immunogenetics: 6:425.
45. Galbraith, R. M., A. L. W. F. Eddleston, R. Williams, et. al. 1976. Enhanced antibody response in active chronic hepatitis in relation to HLA-B8 and HLA-B12 and porta-systemic shunting. Lancet I:390.
46. Scott, B. B., S. M. Rajah, M. L. Swinburne et. al. 1974. HL-A8 and immune response to gluten. Lancet II:374.

47. Cunningham-Rundles, S., C. Cunningham-Rundles, M. S. Pollack, et. al. 1978. Response to wheat antigen in vitro lymphocyte transformation among HLA-B8-positive normal donors. Trans. Proc. 10:977.

48. Bach, J. F., B. Zimgraff, B. Descamps, C. Narak, and P. Jungers. 1975. HLA 1,8 phenotype and HB$_s$ antigenaemia in hemodialysis patients. Lancet II:707.

49. Sasazuki, T., Y. Kohno, I. Iwamoto, and M. Tamimura (1978). Association between an HLA haplotype and low responsiveness to tetanus toxoid in man. Nature 272:359.

50. Spencer, M. J., J. D. Cherry and P. I. Terasaki 1976. HLA-A Antigens and antibody response after influenza A vaccination. New Eng. J. Med. 294:13.

51. DeVries, R. R. P., H. G. Kreeftenberg, H. G. Loggen and J. J. van Road 1977. In vitro immune responsiveness to vaccinia virus and HLA. N. Eng. J. Med. 297:692.

52. Sakane, T., A. D. Steinberg, and I. Green 1978. Studies of immune functions of patients with systemic lupus erythematosus. I. Dysfunction of suppressor T cell activity related to impaired generation of, rather than response to, suppressor cells. Arthritis Rheum. 21:657.

53. James, S., C. O. Elson, E. A. Jones, and W. Strober 1980. Abnormal regulation of immunoglobulin synthesis in vitro in primary biliary cirrhosis. Gastroenterology, in press.

54. Zalko, R. J. and R. L. Dawkins, K. Homes and C. With 1979. Genetic control of suppressor lymphocyte function in myasthenia gravis: relationship of impaired suppressor function to HLA-B8/DRw3 and cold reactive lymphocytotoxic antibodies. Clin. Immunol. and Immunopathol. 14:222.

55. Hodgson, H. J. F., J. R. Wands and K. J. Isselbacher 1977. Suppressor lymphocytes: their role in modulating the immune response in acute and chronic active hepatitis. Gastroenterology 72:1070.

56. Kuntz, M. M., J. B. Innes and M. E. Weksler 1979. The cellular basis of the impaired autologous mixed lymphocyte reaction in patients with systemic lupus erythematosus. J. Clin. Invest. 63:151.

57. James S., C. O. Elson, J. Waggoner, E. A. Jones and W. Strober 1980. Deficiency of the autologous mixed lymphocyte reaction in patients with primary biliary cirrhosis. J. Clin. Invest. In press.

58. Sakane, T. and I. Green 1979. Specificity and suppressor function of T cells responsive to autologous non T cells. J. Immunol. 123:584.

59. Shaw, S., W. E. Biddison 1979. HLA-linked genetic control of the specificity of human cytotoxic T cell responses to influenza virus. J. Exp. Med. 149:565.

60. Biddison, N. E. and S. Shaw 1979. Differences in HLA antigen recognition by human influenza virus-immune cytotoxic T cells. J. Immunol. 122:1705.

61. Geczy, A. F. K. Alexander, H. V. Bashir et. al. 1980. A factor(s) in klebsiella culture filtrates specifically modifies an HLA-B27 associated cell-surface component. Nature 283:782.

Genetic predisposition to allergic disorders: a review

Carl Cohen

Department of Surgery, University of Illinois College of Medicine, Chicago, Illinois

Abstract
    The genetics of atopic diseases cannot be isolated from the mechanisms responsible for the sequence of events from exposure to manifestation of symptoms. Observational data from populations and families for risk evaluation and estimates of mode of inheritance lead to the conclusion that multiple factors are involved. The genes of immunologic significance, e.g., IgE regulation and immune response associated with HLA must be regarded as key parts in the pathogenesis of the disease.

As each new aspect of the science emerges, it is likely to be embraced by a simplistic explanation for whatever is puzzling. Thus allergy – clearly recognized as having concentrations of sufferers in certain families – was investigated for inheritance according to Mendelian genetics. The pendulum swings in theories of the genetics of allergy date from the days of single gene explanations – both dominant and recessive – which lasted from 1916 through the 1930's to the 1950's. Since every attempt to force allergy into a single gene model required abundant use of the fudge factors called penetrance and expressivity, the next logical step was to consider multiple-factor theories. Indeed, additional knowledge has revealed a level of complexity which can be dealt with only if we assume that a number of interactive factors – both genetic and environmental – play a role in the final manifestation of allergic reaction.

The rapid advances which have been made in immunology, including the discovery of IgE, mediators and the putative immune response genes, make it reasonable to assume that complex systems, each of which is poorly understood, result in responses which collectively are called allergy.

Paradoxically, the discovery of IgE and its association with atopic disease attracted investigation and indeed sometimes encouraged some form of fudging (reminiscent of penetrance and expressivity) to force IgE into being the sole responsible factor to allergy. On the other hand, as the importance of the major histocompatibility complex (MHC) genes in cellular recognition of antigens as well as cellular cooperation became evident, stress was naturally placed on an immune response gene being responsible for allergy.

The pendulum has swung again, and a single gene theory has returned. If one wants to be highly sophisticated, one can introduce the immune response gene into some pathway in which a gene controlling IgE is incorporated. In reviewing the genetics of allergy, therefore, one must always be aware of the ever-present desire of research workers to hammer their data into simplistic hypotheses structured to fit the current immunological ideology.

In this review, I will deal with the two approaches: (1) the observational genetics of allergy and then (2) the use of genome differences in the search for mechanisms of allergy. In order to understand the genetics we must start with some generalizations about allergy, mostly drawn from the recently prepared NIAID Task Force Report on Asthma and Other Allergic Disease[1].

The term "allergy" is essentially a general classification for a syndrome which encompasses high variability. For our purposes here it is best to set down some of the characteristics which are generally recognized as constants. Allergy comprises: (1) exposure to the allergen, (2) absorption of the allergen from the mucosal surface, (3) stimulation of the IgE response based on antigen recognition and cellular communication, (4) binding of the IgE to cells, (5) the reaction of the allergen to the bound IgE and, finally, (6) release of chemical mediators from cells and ensuing inflammatory response, resulting in the symptoms of allergy.

Allergens are those antigenic substances which are inhaled, ingested, or injected at appropriate dosage levels (usually relatively low) to stimulate IgE production in susceptible hosts. Marsh[2] suggests that the doses of most inhaled allergens may be less than 1µg/year. The size of the allergen is restricted to its ability to permeate the mucosal membranes of the respiratory tract, with an upper limit possibly of the order of 50,000 daltons. Below this limit, allergens vary widely in their physiocochemical properties (Table 1) and cannot be distinguished as a sub-set of antigens.

An additional condition is imposed by the size of the allergen-containing particle since it may determine the symptoms which develop in susceptible hosts. Particles of greater than 7µ — such as pollen -- are generally trapped in the upper respiratory tract and cause the symptoms of allergic rhinitis (hay fever); particles less than 7µ may reach the lung to stimulate asthmatic symptoms.

Circulating levels of IgE are much lower than the other classes of immunoglobulins, with a median level in unselected individuals of 40-75 units/ml (about 100-180 ng/ml). In selected non-atopic adults, the median level is 21 units/ml[3], and in atopic adults the median is about 200 units/ml[4]. Compared with other immunoglobulin classes, IgE may have a relatively short half-life. This determination is, however, complicated by the facts that the half-life of IgE bound strongly to mast cells and

Table 1. Properties of Some Purified Allergens

Name		Mol. Wt.	pI	No. of Polypeptide chains	Investigator
Rye grass	Rye I	27,000	5.2	1	Marsh
Ragweed	AgE	37,800	5.15	2	King
	Ra3	12,100	8.6	1	Goodfriend
	Ra5	4,900	9.5	1	Goodfriend

basophils is much longer than that of circulating IgE, and that there is exchange between the IgE of the fluid compartment and that bound to tissue. Further important factors are that IgE antibody response is highly T-cell dependent and can be induced by injection of only minute doses of antigen with an appropriate adjuvant in responder animals.

Because several of the multitude of steps in the pathway leading to allergic disease are under genetic control, it is most appropriate to assume multifactorial determination, implying that several genes as well as environmental components are involved. Further, one may assume that each of the genes behaves as a Mendlian factor, and that each is polymorphic. We will consider only those polymorphisms that exist with fairly high frequencies and that represent variants around normal values of responsiveness.

The first polymorphism to be described is that involved in the genetic regulation of IgE formation. As already stated, quantification of the circulating level of IgE by radioimmune assays disclosed that atopic individuals generally have much higher levels than non-allergic persons. Although there is noticeable overlap between the two populations, enough data have been accumulated to accept the idea that high levels are associated with allergy. Genetic analyses by Marsh[6] in 28 families and by Gerrard[7,8] in 173 families indicate that there is a major regulatory locus for IgE levels and that the homozygous recessive maintains a persistently high level of IgE. Both studies report the gene frequency of the two alleles at this locus to be approximately 0.5. It is still not conclusive whether the locus regulates IgE levels directly or whether the levels are secondary manifestations of genetic control of another factor of the many in the cascade leading to allergic symptoms. There are also developmental differences in the IgE level leading to data showing that heritability estimates for adults are different from those of children.

The second critical polymorphic system is derived from the study of tissue transplantation and the development of knowledge about the concentration of important immunologic genes in the chromosomal region called the major histocompatibility complex (MHC). The detection of genes controlling immune response in the guinea pig and the mouse to synthetic polyamino acid antigens led to the concept of the Ir or immune response gene; in the mouse experiments, it soon became clear that the Ir genes are linked to the MHC. Animal studies of the association of the response to allergens to the histocompatibility system by Levine[9] and by Vaz[10] showed that linkage did occur. Studies in atopic human families by Levine[11], Blumenthal[12], and Marsh[13] disclosed allergen Ir genes associated with HLA, the human MHC. Levine's pedigrees indicated that sensitivity to ragweed antigen E was linked to HLA, but no specific allele was singled out. Similarly, Blumenthal found no specific allele in linkage disequilibrium with the Ir gene, although he was able to estimate a recombination distance of 20 centimorgans between the Ir gene and HLA-B. Marsh maintains that the normal level of IgE in an individual cannot be excluded in studies of responsiveness. High serum IgE levels in a person may convert a low responder into a hypersensitive patient; thus the search for the Ir gene for response to allergies is meaningful only in individuals of low IgE phenotype.

A large number of studies on the association of HLA and allergy have been collected by de Weck[14] for inclusion in the conference on HLA and diseases. Tables 2 and 3 are taken from his paper to demonstrate the extent of the surveys and the degree of diversity of the results.

Two other systems which play a role in the allergic response are the complement system and the Hageman factor systems. Both involve several independent genes, and several of these have been shown to be polymorphic. There is no hard evidence yet for the role that these polymorphisms play in

Table 2. Association between HLA and Atopic Disease (modified from de Weck[14])

	Author	HLA Association	p value
A. Atopic Dermatitis	Krain	↑A3,A9	.05
	Turner	↑A1,B8	.02
	Hoshino	↑B5	.05
	Ohkido	↑B12	Not given
	Ohkido	↑BW40	.01
	Goudemand	↑BW35	.01
	Scholz	None	—
B. Bronchial Asthma	Thorsby	↑A1,B8	.05
		↑A2,B8	.05
	Rachelefsky	↑A2,↓B8	Not given
	Morris	↑A1	.02
		↑B8	.01
		↑B12	.02

Table 3. Association between HLA and Response to Purified Allergens (modified from de Weck[14])

Allergen	Type of Study	Author	HLA Association	p Value
AgE	Population	Marsh	–	–
Ra5	"	Marsh	↑B7	.03
Ra5	"	Goodfriend	↑B7	.01
Ra3	"(low-IgE)	Marsh	↑A2	.04
	"	"	↑B12	.07
	"	"	↑A3	–
Rye I	"(low-IgE)	"	↑B8	.005
			↑A1,B8	.007
AgE	Family	Levine	Family haplo.	
AgE	"	Blumenthal	"	
AgE	"	Yoo	"	
AgE	"	Black[15]	No association	
Ra3	"	"	"	
Ra5	"	"	"	
Rye I	"	"	"	

producing the variability in response of the atopic patient. The polymorphism of the complement system, although of great significance in
several disease states, has not yet been associated with atopic disease.
The Hageman factor system has not been exploited for studies of genetic
polymorphism.

I wish to conclude with an examination of the general problems
existent in attempt to draw simplistic conclusions from data which suggest
the association of an HLA allele with atopic diseases.

Although there may be strong associations between a particular factor and the disease in question (atopy), the associations are rarely absolute. Some of the possible causes for this inconsistency bear consideration for they indicate how we must treat our multiple factor model. The most important basis for inconsistency is the fact that the HLA allele which is highly associated may not be the gene directly involved in the disease process but may be a marker for a gene or genes linked to it. The strength of the association of the HLA allele with the disease may be dependent on the linkage disequilibrium or the interdependence between the HLA allele and the gene more directly associated with the manifestation of the allergy. In different populations it is quite possible that the disequilibrium may be between the disease-associated gene and different MHC genes, leading to regional, ethnic or racial differences in the association.

In atopy, an important factor which may be responsible for lack of uniform association is the very heterogeneous manifestation of response. Although a variety of clinical syndromes are loosely classified as atopy, we cannot overlook the fact that we are dealing with a potpourri of diseases which may have different pathways -- perhaps not greatly different, but different -- between stimulus and manifestations. Where a single step in a pathway is changed the gene responsible for the character of that step may have a different association or perhaps no obvious association at all. Perhaps these different HLA associations can be used for classification of allergic patients, which may ultimately result in separation of a single disease which has variability into two or more distinct groups.

Since we are using HLA genes as markers and in some ways the HLA system is still engendering a significant amount of investigation, particularly in defining specificities or target cells of the serological typing reagents, the HLA system is still changing. The recognition that the MHC has several loci arranged in linear order with genetic distances

between them makes it conceivable there are still undetected — but
potentially detectable — loci to be discovered. Each new locus has the
potential of being a better marker because of the shorter distances
between the actual disease-controlling gene and the HLA gene or stronger
linkage disequilibrium.

Actually the multiple factor hypothesis forbids the restriction
of a complex series of interactions between several genes and the rest of
the intrinsic and extrinsic environment to the action of one or two loci.
The genetic uniqueness of practically every individual is a major
contributor to the heterogeneity in the disease collection called atopy
and the finding of strong consistent association is not going to be a
common event. Nor should we be too forceful in requiring that there be
an association between HLA allele and atopy.

The finding that in a particular family there is an association
between hypersensitivity and a particular haplotype but that different
haplotypes are involved in other families indicates that the HLA gene
may be linked to an essential gene for atopic manifestation but that the
genes are not in linkage disequilibrium nor are we dealing with multiple
roles of a single gene. The search for pedigrees which prove a point is
dangerous unless the number of pedigrees searched and discarded is
included in the data.

CONCLUSION

In conclusion, I have emphasized the complex multifactorial nature
of atopic allergy. All attempts to fit this disease into single-
gene inheritance by application of fudge factors such as variable
penetrance and expressivity merely serve to confuse the issue. Further
approaches toward understanding the complex genetics of this disease
should take a balanced view of our current understanding of the roles of
IgE, HLA and cellular regulation of the immune response, as well as of

important environmentral factors. One should also be open to new

discoveries of factors which might influence the immunological and

pharmacological manifestations of this disease.

REFERENCES

1. NIAID Task Force Report on Asthma and Other Allergic Diseases.
1979. NIH Publication 79-387.
2. Marsh, D.G. and W.B. Bias. 1976. Atopic Allergy: A Model for
Studying the Genetics of Immune Response in Man. Birth Defects: Original
Article Series 12: 223-237.
3. Nye, L., T.G. Merrit, J. Landon, and R.J. White. 1975. A detailed
investigation of circulating IgE levels in a normal population. Clinical
Allergy 5: 13-24.
4. Marsh, D.G., and W.B. Bias. 1977. Basal serum IgE levels and HLA
frequencies in allergic subjects: I. Studies with ragweed allergen Ra3.
Immunogenetics 5: 217-233.
5. Cohen, C. 1974. Genetic Aspects of Allergy. The Med. Clin. of N.
Amer. 15(1): 25-42.
6. Marsh, D.G., W.B. Bias, and K. Ishizaka. 1974. Genetic control of
basal serum immunoglobulin E level and its effect on specific reaginic
sensitivity. Proc. Nat. Acad. Sci. (Wash.) 71: 3588-3592.
7. Gerrard, J.W., S. Horne, P. Vickers, J.W.A. MacKenzie, N. Goluboff,
J.Z. Garson, and C. Maningas. 1974. Serum IgE levels in parents and
children. J. Pediatrics 85: 660-663.
8. Gerrard, J.W., D.C. Rao, and N.E. Morton. 1978. A genetic study of
immunoglobulin E. Am. J. Hum. Genet. 30(1): 46-58.
9. Levine, B.B. and N.M. Vaz, 1970. Effect of combinations of inbred
production in the mouse: A potential mouse model for immune aspects of
human atopic allergy. Int. Arch. Allergy 39: 156-171.
10. Vaz, N.M. and B.B. Levine. 1970. Immune Reponses of inbred
mice to repeated low doses of antigens: relationship to histocompatibility (H-2) type. Science 168: 852-854.
11. Levin, B.B., R.H. Stember, and M. Fotino. 1972. Ragweed hayfever:
genetic control and linkage to HL-A haplotypes. Science 178: 1201-1203.
12. Blumenthal, M.N., D.B. Amos, H. Noreen, N.R. Mendell and E.F.
Yunis. 1979. Genetic mapping of Ir locus in man: linkage to second
locus of HL-A. Science 184: 1301-1303.
13. Marsh, D.G., S.H. Hsu and W.B. Bias. 1972. Test of Association
between HL-A histocompatibility antigens and immediate hypersensitivity
reactions to highly purified allergens in man. J. Allergy 49: 124-125.
14. deWeck, A.L. 1977. HLA and Allergy. In Monographs in allergy
11: 3-18.
15. Black, P.L., D.G. Marsh, F. Jarrett, G.J. Delespesse and W.B. Bias.
1976. Family studies of association between HLA and specific immune
responses to highly purified pollen allergens. Immunogenetics
3: 349-368.

SESSION II

Summary of Discussion

Discussion centered around the continuing need for better characterization of human HLA-D region genes, gene products and their involvement in
the immune response. The relative usefulness of monoclonal antibodies,
conventional D-"locus" homozygous typing cells and PLT cell lines (Bach)
for defining D-region specificities was indicated. Several discussants
favored the serologic approach to typing of D-region specificities. It was
the consensus that though serologic analysis does have problems, advances
are expected in the near future as monoclonal antibodies which recognize
specific alloantigens are developed. However, at present, only species-
specific antibodies are readily available.

One opinion expressed was that while the use of cultured PLT cells over
serologic methods of DR typing was not favored, it was thought that cloned
PLT cells would provide much needed complementary information to that
obtained with the use of DR typing sera in view of the complexity of the
human D region. It was further pointed out that cloning of PLT cells
presently has an advantage in that cells of desired specificity could be
selected and by appropriate culture methods high yields could be obtained
(e.g., 10^9 cells within seven weeks).

Consideration was given to conventional typing for D-locus antigens
using homozygous typing cells. This was noted to be a "messy" system in
regard to precise definition of D specificities; attempts to gain a clear

distinction between the presence or absence of a particular D-locus antigen often failed. The use of cultured D-homozygous typing cells was found to be even more difficult in view of the autoreactivity expressed by many of these cellular elements. The thought was expressed that cultured PLT typing cells would therefore probably replace the currently used homozygous typing cells. In the subsequent discussion it was stressed that despite problems with typing using D-homozygous cells, they were particularly useful as reagents for the biochemical analysis of HLA-D antigens. However, in such cases it should be assured that all cells used are completely homozygous in regard to HLA, i.e., complete identity for the entire HLA complex on both chromosomes, a finding that might occur in the offspring of first-cousin matings.

It was then pointed out that continuing search for sera having specificity for particular T cell differentiation antigens in man could be especially useful. Work was cited to emphasize the analytic power of mouse monoclonal antibodies against particular T cell antigens[1,2]. Similar reagents directed against antigens expressed on natural killer (NK) cells could also serve a useful purpose in dissecting the genetics of this system.

The high degree of complexity of the human D region was emphasized throughout the discussion. Dissection of this complexity appears to be a key problem in elucidating the genetics of human immune responses especially with regard to relating human studies to those performed in mouse models.

In opening the discussion on HLA and ocular disease, the association of B27 with ankylosing spondylitis and related rheumatic diseases was noted. In such disorders, as well as in histoplasmosis and Behcet's syndrome, eye involvement had usually been studied only as a secondary issue to other symptoms. In order to understand possible unique genetic factors in individuals having ocular involvement, investigation should consider those subsets of patients manifesting eye symptoms and those who do not. It is unfortunate that D-locus typing has generally not been performed in the case of ocular diseases but this should certainly be pursued in view of the strong D-locus associations found for many other disorders.

An interesting study was described noting the prevalence of A1, B8 phenotype in American blacks affected by anterior uveitis. In such situations there is a marked association particularly with B8, surprisingly not yet demonstrated in Caucasians. Clarification is needed in view of the much stronger association of B8 with autoimmune disease in whites than in the black population in the U.S.

Particular emphasis was placed upon the association between B8 and Dw3 and a wide variety of autoimmune diseases and diseases with suspected autoimmune components, e.g., gluten-sensitive enteropathy. Such associations are of interest to ophthalmologists in view of the occurrence of a number of putative autoimmune diseases of the eye. It was pointed out that all autoimmune diseases may share a common mechanism associated with particular allele(s) of gene(s) mapping within HLA and in linkage disequilibrium with the B8-Dw3 haplotype. However, to be emphasized is the probable presence of additional genes unique for the disease in question, which might be linked or not linked to the HLA system. In subsequent discussion, the belief was expressed that it was important to determine the reason why women are more susceptible than men to autoimmune disease. In pertinent work on NZB mice[3] it was pointed out that this model may provide evidence for sex-associated hormonal factors rather than x-linked genes influencing the expression of autoimmune disease.

Commented upon were the rather low values for the "relative risk" for several of these discussed diseases pointing to the possibility that such low values could conceivably be due to such trivial explanations as the "founder effects" or population migrations. However, on the whole, the consistent association of most autoimmune diseases with B8 and Dw3 present a rather coherent story in most people's opinions making such explanations unlikely. In response to a question as to whether severity of disease might be more strongly associated with particular HLA specificities, the example of more persistent antithyroid antibody in B8 positive patients with Grave's disease was cited[4].

Then discussed were interesting reported negative associations between a number of autoimmune diseases and the presence of B7, D(R)w2 phenotypes[4]. In recent data from both Minnesota and Copenhagen relating to a total of some 220 patients with insulin dependent (juvenile onset) diabetes not one case of Dw2 or DRw2 have been found even though the phenotypic frequencies of these related specificities are about 20 percent in normal Caucasian populations. Thus, D(R)w2 may be associated with resistance to certain diseases having an autoimmune component. Commented upon was another group of diseases including multiple sclerosis and Goodpasture's syndrome, where D(R)w2 was elevated[4], suggesting the possibility of increased suscepti-bility to viruses in patients with this phenotype. To be considered, however, is the fact of several HLA associations with diseases that have no apparent immunologic component,[4] e.g., hemochromotosis with HLA-3. Therefore, it is important to have a broader look than one simply directed to putative immune components in evaluating HLA associations.

Overall there was sentiment that much is to be learned about autoimmune diseases on both genetic and nongenetic levels. A present view holds that genes in linkage disequilibrium with the B8, Dw3 haplotype appear to be a necessary but not sufficient condition for the expression of autoimmune diseases in many patients.

In considering the genetic predisposition to allergic disorders, the multifactorial determination of atopic disease was emphasized. Genetic factors including an IgE-regulating gene not linked to HLA have been described as well as a probable role for HLA linked Ir genes similar to those described in the mouse. Additionally, environmental factors are undoubtedly as important in allergy as in other diseases. While significant associations have been found between sensitivity to specific highly purified allergens and the presence of particular HLA types, demonstration of genetic linkage in families between HLA and specific Ir genes has so far not been convincing. Despite some expressed skepticism, statistical data strongly indicate the involvement of major genetic factors controlling the expression of atopic disease[5]. At a recent workshop on the genetics of IgE all available data suggested that there is a major gene regulation of the IgE level and that this gene may be a major determinant of specific IgE responsiveness.

In addition to genetic factors, subsequent discussion brought forth mention of recent unpublished work (Marsh) demonstrating the overall ability to generate an IgE response to any complex antigen (including heterogenous material such as house dust) associated with the A1, B8, Dw3 phenotype. This was considered to be of particular interest in view of the association of B8 and Dw3 with autoimmune disease discussed earlier and of the A1, B8 haplotype with rejection of kidney transplants[6,7]. Believed to becoming increasingly clear is the concept that generalized immune hyper-responsiveness, such as seen in autoimmune disease, atopic allergy and transplant rejection, is associated with the most common Caucasian haplotype, A1, B8, Dw3.

These data suggest that the conventional view of specific Ir genes in disease needs to be re-evaluated. Perhaps as expressed by one discussant, the (A1), B8, Dw3 haplotype may be in linkage disequilibrium with genes involved in general mechanisms of immune regulation. Another possibility may be the view that perhaps "specific" Ir genes do not really have the degree of specificity hitherto believed. In regard to ocular disease, the precise mechanism of genetic factors associated with B27 and the B8, Dw3

phenotypes deserve especial attention in future investigations.

REFERENCES

1. Reinherz, E. L., P. C. Kung, J. M. Pesando, J. Ritz, G. Goldstein, and S. F. Schlossman. 1979. Ia determinants on human T-cell subsets defined by monoclonal antibody: Activation stimuli required for expression. J. Exp. Med. 150: 1472.
2. Reinherz, E. L., P. C. Kung, G. Goldstein, and S. F. Schlossman. 1979. Separation of functional subsets of human T cells by monoclonal antibody. Proc. Natl. Acad. Sci. 78: 4061.
3. Raveche, E. S., J. H. Tjio, and A. D. Steinberg. 1979. Genetics of studies in NZB mice. III. Induced anti-nucleic acid antibody production. J. Immunol. 122: 1454.
4. Ryder, L. P., E. Anderson, and A. Svejgaard. 1979. HLA and disease registry, Third Report. Munksgaard, Copenhagen.
5. Marsh, D. G., and W. B. Bias. 1978. The genetics of atopic disease. In Immunological diseases (3rd edition) Chapter 45. Edited by M. Samter. Little, Brown and Company, Boston, P. 819.
6. Kissmeyer-Nielsen, F. et al. 1971. Scanditransplant: preliminary report of a kidney exchange program. Transpl. Proc. 3: 1019.
7. Mickey, M. R., M. Kreisler, E. D. Albert, N. Tanaka, and P. I Terasaki. 1971. Analysis of HLA incompatibility in human renal transplants. Tissue Antigens 1: 57.

SESSION III

IMMUNOLOGY OF TISSUE TRANSPLANTATION

Moderator: Arthur M. Silverstein

Renal transplantation: cumulative influence of combined risk factors

Richard L.Simmons, Bruce G.Sommer, David E.R.Sutherland, Richard J.Howard and John S. Najarian

Department of Surgery, University of Minnesota, Minneapolis, Minnesota 55455

ABSTRACT

Seven hundred sixty-seven primary renal allografts from a single center were divided into subgroups according to combinations of several major risk factors: donor source and histocompatibility match, age and presence or absence of diabetes. The relative effect of diabetes on patient and graft survival decreased as histocompatibility differences increased. The influence of recipient age, however, dramatically decreased as histocompatibility differences decreased. In all groups donor source and histocompatibility match had the strongest relative effect in determining subsequent 2-year patient and graft survival.

INTRODUCTION

Analysis of transplant patient populations according to single risk factors is useful in determining the general influence of each factor on patient and graft functional survival.[1] We have previously reported the effect of recipient age[2], donor source[3-5], and the presence or absence of recipient diabetes[6,7] as single factors influencing recipient and graft survival in renal transplant patients. For the individual patient, however, risk factors occur in various combinations. We divided recipients of primary renal transplants into multiple groups according to all possible combinations of these three major risk factors, and calculated patient survival and graft function following renal transplantation. The present study isolates subgroups of patients within "high-risk" groups with graft and recipient survival differing from the expected.

MATERIALS AND METHODS

The results in 767 consecutive recipients of first renal transplants performed between January 1, 1968 and September 1, 1977 and followed through March 1, 1978 were analyzed. Our standard operative technique and immunosuppressive regimen have been previously described.[8] Tissue typing and cross-matching were performed in our immunology laboratory as previously described[9] For the purposes of this analysis, the match between donor and recipient was assessed according to the HLA antigens identified at the A and B loci. The

patients were categorized according to the combinations of three main risk
factors: donor source and histocompatibility match; presence or absence of
diabetes; and age ($\leq$ 16 years old, 17 to 49 years old, and $\geq$ 50 years old).

The comparisons made in this analysis were survival of the patients and
functional survival of the transplanted kidneys. All causes of death, even
death on dialysis following graft loss, and all causes of loss of kidney function were included in the analysis. Patient and graft survival in all
groups was calculated by standard actuarial techniques.[10] The results for
all groups consisting of at least 20 patients at 2 years after transplantation are given in the tables. The differences in 2-year survival rates were
compared by utilizing a t test for differences of proportions. The 0.05
level of significance was used to determine statistically significant differences.

RESULTS

Patient and graft survival at 2 years for all subgroups containing at
least 20 patients are tabulated in Table 1. The groups have been listed in
order of decreasing patient survival. Non-diabetic recipients of intermediate age who receive renal allografts from HLA-identical sibling donors have
the best survival and graft function, while patients $\geq$ 50 years old who receive poorly matched cadaver kidneys do the least well. Although these results are expected from previous analyses of individual risk factors, the
relative position of some combinations between these two extremes are informative. Some patients previously considered to be at high risk actually have
better survival than those not previously considered in a high-risk category.
For example, diabetic children of intermediate age receiving grafts from parental donors do better than nondiabetic recipients of young or intermediate
age receiving grafts from poorly matched cadaver donors. To aid the interpretation of the data, we have analyzed each risk factor controlling for the
other variables.

Effect of age. Table 2 shows the effect of the recipient's age on patient survival and graft function when the donor source and the metabolic
status of the recipient are controlled. The majority of our diabetic patients
are between 17 and 49 years old, and thus not enough diabetic patients are
available in other age categories for comparison. There is a definite trend
toward less satisfactory results as ages increase. However, the influence of
recipient age is minimized as histocompatibility is increased between the
donor and recipient; for instance, in nondiabetic patients $\geq$ 50 years old,
survival can be increased from 47% with $\leq$ 1 antigen matched cadaver grafts to
91% if the kidney is donated from a related child.

Table 1. Two-year cumulative patient and graft survival rates in recipients of primary renal transplants according to combined risk factors

Group[a]	Donor source	Recipient status	Recipient age (years)	Patient survival	P<0.05[b] versus groups	Graft function	P<0.05[b] versus groups
1	HLA-ID[c] sibling	Nondiabetic sibling	17-49	98	7-17 9-17	92	4,5,7 9-17
2	Related child	Nondiabetic parent	17-49	94	11-17	84	7,11,12 14-17
3	Related child	Nondiabetic parent	>50	91	11-14 16,17	79	7,12,15 17
4	Related parent	Nondiabetic child	<16	90	11-14 16,17	66	1,6,17
5	HLA non-ID sibling	Nondiabetic sibling	17-49	89	11-14 16,17	73	1,12,17
6	HLA-ID sibling	Diabetic sibling	17-49	87	12,14 16,17	86	7,11-17
7	CAD>2 Ag Match[d]	Nondiabetic	17-49	84	1,14,17	62	1-3,6,8 17
8	Related parent	Diabetic child	17-49	82	1,17	81	7,11,12 15,17
9	Related parent	Nondiabetic child	17-49	81	1,17	69	1,17
10	Distant- ly related	Nondiabetic distantly related	17-49	72	1,17	60	1,17
11	CAD>2 Ag match	Diabetic	17-49	72	1-5,17	60	1,2,6, 8,17
12	CAD<1 Ag match	Nondiabetic	17-49	70	1-6,17	57	1-3,5,6 8,17
13	CAD<1 Ag match	Nondiabetic	<16	70	1-5,17	62	1,6,17
14	HLA non-ID sibling	Diabetic sibling	17-49	69	1-7,17	62	1,2,6 17
15	CAD<1 Ag match	Diabetic	17-49	67	1-2,17	52	1-3,6, 8,17
16	CAD>2 Ag match	Nondiabetic	>50	60	1-6,17	55	1,2,6 17
17	CAD<1 Ag match	Nondiabetic	>50	47	1-15	36	1-16

[a] All groups contain at least 20 patients at 2 years.
[b] P>0.05 versus all other groups.
[c] ID, identical; CAD, cadaver
[d] A and B loci only.

Effect of diabetes. Table 3 shows the effect of recipient diabetes on patient and graft survival when age and donor source are controlled. When histocompatibility differences are at a minimum (HLA-identical sibling donors), the recipient pays a definite penalty for being diabetic; patient survival is 11% less and graft survival is 6% less than that of nondiabetic

Table 2. Effect of age on 2-year cumulative patient and graft survival rates when donor source and the presence or absence of diabetes are controlled

Group[a]	Recipient age (years)		Presence or absence of diabetes	Survival	
				Patient	Graft
2	17-49	Child	Nondiabetic	94	84
3	>50			91	79
4	<16	Parent	Nondiabetic	90	66
9	17-49			81	69
7	17-49	CAD[b] >2 Ag match	Nondiabetic	84	62
16	>50			60	55
13	<16	CAD <1 Ag match	Nondiabetic	70	62
12	17-49			70	57
17	>50			47	36

[a]Refer to Table 1 for P.
[b]CAD, cadaver

Table 3. Effect of diabetes mellitus on 2-year cumulative patient and graft survival rates when recipient age and donor source are controlled

Group[a]	Presence or absence of diabetes	Donor source	Recipient age (years)	Survival	
				Patient	Graft
1	Nondiabetic	HLA-ID[b] Sibling	17-49	98	92
6	Diabetic			87	86
5	Nondiabetic	HLA non-ID Sibling	17-49	89	73
14	Diabetic			69	62
9	Nondiabetic	Parent	17-49	81	69
8	Diabetic			82	81
7	Nondiabetic	CAD > 2 Ag match	17-49	84	62
11	Diabetic			72	60
12	Nondiabetic	CAD < 1 Ag match	17-49	70	57
15	Diabetic			67	52

[a]Refer to Table 1 for P.
[b]ID, identical; CAD, cadaver.

patients. However, in general, the differences in survival between diabetic and nondiabetic patients are minimized as histocompatibility differences decrease between the donor and recipient. There is essentially no difference in patient and graft survival between diabetics and nondiabetics receiving grafts from cadaver donors matched for <1 HLA antigen with the recipient.

Effect of donor source. Table 4 shows the relative effect of donor

Table 4. Effect of donor source of 2-year cumulative patient and graft survival rates when recipient age and the presence or absence of diabetes are controlled.

Group[a]	Donor source	Recipient age (years)	Presence or absence of diabetes	Survival Patient	Graft
1	HLA-ID[b] Sibling	17-49	Nondiabetic	98	92
2	Related child			94	84
5	HLA non-ID sibling			89	73
9	Related parent			81	69
10	Distantly related			72	60
7	CAD $\geq$ 2 Ag match	17-49	Nondiabetic	84	62
12	CAD $\leq$ 1 Ag match			70	57
6	HLA-ID Sibling	17-49	Diabetic	87	86
8	Related parent			82	81
14	HLA non-ID sibling			69	62
11	CAD $\geq$ 2 Ag match	17-49	Diabetic	72	60
15	CAD $\leq$ 1 Ag match			67	52
3	Related parent	$\geq$50	Nondiabetic	91	79
16	CAD $\geq$ 2 Ag match			60	55
17	CAD $\leq$ 1 Ag match			47	36

[a] Refer to Table 1 for P.
[b] ID, Identical; CAD, cadaver

source on patient and graft survival when age and presence or absence of diabetes are controlled. Increasing histocompatibility differences between the donor and recipient decrease patient and graft survival, regardless of the age or metabolic status of the patient. In all age categories and in both diabetics and nondiabetics, recipients receiving grafts from HLA-identical siblings have an advantage over recipients receiving poorly matched cadaveric grafts. Conversely, in recipients of poorly matched cadaver kidneys ($\leq$1 HLA antigen shared) the results are equally poor in all age categories and in both diabetics and nondiabetics.

DISCUSSION

This analysis of 767 consecutive primary renal transplants generally confirms previous conclusions concerning the individual influence of three basic risk factors. Transplantation is less successful in patients with diabetes, but not in all subcategories. Older patients do worse than younger patients, but there are exceptions. Patients receiving kidneys from HLA-identical sibling donors generally do better than patients without such donors, but other categories can do almost as well.

The effects of the three risk factors changes according to their combination. For example, the relative effect of recipient diabetes or older age changes as histocompatibility differences change. Diabetes manifests itself as a major risk factor when histocompatibility effects are at a minimum; however, this effect decreases as histocompatibility differences between the donor and recipient are decreased. Age, on the other hand, appears to have little effect on patient and graft survival when histocompatibility differences are small. However, recipient age is a high-risk factor when histocompatibility differences between the donor and recipient are increased. Since neither age nor the presence or absence of recipient diabetes can be altered prior to transplantation, the importance of selecting the best donor is emphasized. Graft source can often be manipulated to change a patient from a high risk to an average or low-risk category, increasing the success rate of renal transplantation.

Although transplants from HLA-identical sibling donors to nondiabetic recipients are the most successful, results with renal grafts from children to nondiabetic parents in the intermediate age group are almost as good at 2 years after transplantation. In another example, kidneys transplanted from well matched cadaver donors results in patient and graft survival that is similar to that obtained using kidneys from HLA-nonidentical related donors. Nevertheless, even when an HLA-identical sibling is not available as a donor, our present policy is to transplant kidneys from HLA-nonidentical related donors whenever possible, rather than place the patient on a waiting list for cadaver kidney transplantation. Most patients must wait several months before a well matched cadaver graft is found. More importantly, because of the limited availability of cadaver organs, we continue to use related donors from the immediate family whenever possible. If this policy is not followed, many patients will not receive transplants.

A very high-risk group appears to be the older patient who receives a poorly matched cadaver kidney. However, age itself does not automatically place the recipient in a high-risk category. Patient and graft survival are dramatically improved in this group if a related donor kidney (usually from a child) is utilized.

One point that should be noted is that in some categories patient and graft survival rates differ by only a small percentage. These results may mean that emphasis is placed on salvaging failing grafts at the expense of patient survival. However, this trend is most pronounced in the diabetic population, and may be unavoidable in these patients. In diabetics, death, particularly from cardiovascular disease, is a frequent cause of graft loss. In addition, when graft loss occurs for other reasons in the diabetic patient, long-term survival on dialysis is poor.[6,7]

It is apparent that there are certain limitations to a study which attempts to simultaneously analyze combinations of several factors. Statistical analysis of subpopulations is impaired because of insufficient numbers of patient in some subgroups, and in some instances only trends can be noted. However, the differences in survival between certain groups are very large, and should not be ignored simply because the number of patients in the group are too small for a P of <0.05 to be reached.

In summary, this method of analysis shows that donor source and HLA match are more important than presence or absence of diabetes or age in predicting patient and graft functional survival. An analysis of this type can be used to indicate to an individual patient, pretransplant, the expected prognosis for survival and graft function according to age, presence or absence of diabetes, and donor sources available.

REFERENCES

1. Salvatierra, O., A.J. Feduska, K.C. Cochrum, et al. 1977. Ann. Surg. 186:424.
2. Kjellstrand, C.M., J.R. Shideman, R.E. Lynch, et al. 1976. Geriatrics 31:65.
3. Simmons, R.L., E.J. Thompson, C.M. Kjellstrand, et al. 1976. Lancet 1: 321.
4. Simmons, R.L., E.J. Van Hook, E.J. Yunis, et al. 1977. Ann. Surg. 185: 196.
5. Simmons, R.L., E.J. Thompson, E.J. Yunis, et al. 1977.Am. J. Med. 62:234.
6. Sutherland, D.E.R., C.M. Kjellstrand, R.L. Simmons, et al. 1976. Minn. Med. 59:766.
7. Najarian, J.S., D.E.R. Sutherland, R.L. Simmons, et al. 1977. Surg. Gynecol. Obstet. 144:682.
8. Simmons, R.L., C.M. Kjellstrand, J.S. Najarian. 1972. p. 445 In Najarian, J.S., Simmons, R.L. (eds), Transplantation. Lea and Febiger, Philadelphia.
9. Callender, C.O., R.L. Simmons, E.J. Yunis, et al. 1974. Surgery 76:573.
10. Merrell, M., L.E. Shulman. 1955. J. Chronic Dis. 1:12.

Allografts of cultured organs

Richard Hong, M.D.

Departments of Pediatrics and Medical Microbiology, University of Wisconsin Clinical Science Center, Madison, Wisconsin

ABSTRACT

Organ culture can permit acceptance of allografts between strains of strong histocompatibility differences. The best results to date have been observed with thyroid grafts in mice and thymus grafts in mouse and man. In these situations, excellent functional reconstitution is seen. Allograft acceptance is due to loss of passenger leukocytes which may uniquely provide a special set of alloantigens (LD) which are necessary for complete sensitization of the recipient. In addition to restoration, thymus transplantation into athymic mice has the unique ability to induce tolerance for the alloantigens of the donor. This creates a remarkable situation in which an animal is tolerant of two sets of alloantigens, self and histoincompatible thymus donor.

INTRODUCTION

In 1967, Jacobs and Huseby[1] demonstrated that following short term maintenance in organ culture various tumors could be successfully transplanted across major histocompatibility differences. Subsequently, it was shown that organ culture allowed successful allograft transplantation of normal ovary[2,3], thyroid[4], pancreatic islet cells[5], parathyroids[6] and thymus[7]. In addition, thymus epithelial monolayers have been developed and transplanted[8,9]. The culture technique is very effective and essentially permanent engraftment (> 70 days) has been recorded for mouse thyroid allografts[4]. Even xenografts are accepted[10].

ORGAN CULTURE TECHNIQUES

The techniques employed are rather similar except for the monolayers. Very small organs such as mouse thyroids are cultured intact, but otherwise the tissues are minced or cut into small (approximately 2 mm in diameter) fragments. They are floated or supported on the surface of the culture medium, the choice of which seems not critical. We favor Ham's F-12 for our thymic cultures, but no systemized study has been made of the various merits of different media. Waymouth's medium is popular for thymus epithelium monolayer culture as it does not support lymphocytes[11]. Fetal calf serum or homologous serum (usually 10%) is added for support. The time of culture varies from 48 hours to several weeks.

Enzyme disruption has been used to set up thymic monolayer cultures[8,12]. The medium is supplemented with 30% fetal calf serum to inhibit fibroblast overgrowth. An interesting problem unique to thymic monolayers is the development of autodestructive cytotoxic T cells[11]. For this reason, thymocytes must be removed repeatedly during the initial period of culture.

Others have developed monolayers from explants of small fragments[11,13,14,15]. The method by which the monolayer is developed controls greatly the predominant cell type of the monolayer (J. Jones, personal communication).

TRANSPLANTATION

For most of the tissues employed, the site of transplant seems irrelevant as long as adequate vascularization occurs. Humoral products secreted into the blood stream can reconstitute deficiency states. One unconfirmed report asserts that an intraadrenal transplant of rat parathyroid will function when intramuscular transplants do not[16]. Intraperitoneal, sub-fascial and sub-renal capsule sites have been employed with success. In the case of cultured thymus transplants, a few intraperitoneal transplants have been performed, but we prefer the renal capsule in nude mice and the intramuscular site in man. The intramuscular transplant can be easily biopsied and a judgment of the success of engraftment made (Fig. 1). Intraabdominal transplants in man may be associated with neoplasms[17].

EFFECTS OF CULTURE

Save for thymic epithelial monolayers, all cultured transplants to date have involved culture of organ fragments. In vitro assessment of the cultured fragments has shown that pancreatic islets and thymic fragments demonstrate evidence for some physiologic capability for periods varying from seven to eighteen days[18,19]. Thyroid pieces, cultured for as long as twenty-six days can still restore endocrine function in vivo[20]. As assessed by chemotaxis experiments, thymic fragment cultures

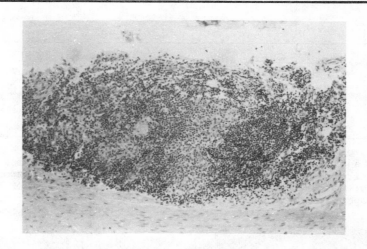

Figure 1. Cultured thymus transplanted into child with severe combined immunodeficiency. Biopsy 4 months later is rich in lymphocytes. Original X 63.

are functional for nine to ten days and marked changes in the character of the cells attracted occur thereafter[19].

In Figure 2 and Table I are shown typical results of incubating peripheral blood or bone marrow mononuclear cells with

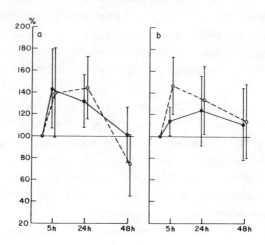

Figure 2. Incubation of peripheral blood mononuclear cells with cultured thymic fragments. a) Culture for 7 days. b) Culture for 19 days. Ordinate shows percent increase in response and abcissa shows hours of incubation. Phytohemagglutinin stimulation.

TABLE I

Stimulus

THYMUS	BONE MARROW	PHA	CON A	NONE
-	Pt	5664 + 299	1889 + 143	337 + 75
Pt	Pt	7999 + 672	2494 + 194	517 + 118
Normal	Pt	19518 + 1293	12818 + 1614	800 + 152
Normal	Normal	24503 + 899	17335 + 659	1528 + 195

Results of incubation of normal and patient bone marrow with normal and patient (Pt) cultured thymus. Source of thymus or bone marrow shown in columns at left. Proliferative response (in cpm) to phytohemagglutinin (PHA), Concanavalin A (CON A) or no mitogen is shown.

cultured thymic fragments. It can be seen that cells predestined for thymic differentiation can be influenced in vitro as an indicator of thymic or mononuclear cell capability. Similar results have been reported by others[21,22].

In humans, a morphologically normal thymus transplant has been recovered in a patient who showed clinical and laboratory evidence for T cell reconstitution; the transplant had been in culture for sixteen days. Thyroid, parathyroid and islet cell transplants secrete humoral substances and the question of a 3-dimensional requirement for complete biological restitution is less significant in these cases. For thymus transplants however, inward migration of bone marrow stem cells with subsequent cell-cell interaction is required and it is conceivable that spatial needs must be fulfilled. Thus, it may not be possible for thymic monolayers to effect adequate T cell reconstitution. In a previous study, rat epithelial monolayer transplants did not become lymphoid[12]. Jordan et al[9], however, report epithelio-lymphoid structures following transplantation of twenty-eight day old monolayer cultures. As the transplantation was performed in syngeneic thymus bearing normals, no effects on functional reconstitution could be measured.

The function of cultured allogeneic transplants is variable. Pancreatic and thyroid grafts seem to restore completely chemically or surgically induced deficiencies[4,5]. Thymus transplants completely restore congenitally athymic nuce mice[23].

Ovarian and parathyroid grafts function for prolonged periods, but permanent acceptance has not as yet been shown. In man, cultured thymic transplants have been shown to restore both T and B cell functions, even to the extent of forming specific antibody following virus infections[24].

PASSENGER LEUKOCYTE CONCEPT

The acceptance of the graft is most likely due to the loss of "passenger leukocytes" during the culture period. As early as 1957, Snell[25] suggested that donor lymphocytes passively carried over in a graft were particularly effective in stimulating allograft immunity. A number of studies subsequent to that time confirmed this notion (reviewed by Billingham[26]). The support for this concept can be briefly summarized thus:

1) In a local graft versus host reaction (skin or kidney) the host must deliver lymphoid cells to the area of graft inoculum or the reaction will not occur. In other words, injected cytotoxic T killer cells fail to react against surrounding alloantigen unless host leukocytes are also present[26].

2) A kidney returned to the donor after a period of sojourn into an allogeneic host was rejected, i.e., an animal could be made to reject his own kidney. Apparently, host cells infiltrate the organ and serve as the target for the rejection[26].

Further insight into the mechanism was provided by Talmage et al who showed that injection of peritoneal exudate cells (PEC) of donor type caused prompt rejection of a previously accepted cultured thyroid graft[27]. This study confirmed that acceptance was not on the basis of tolerance, but rather incomplete sensitization, a deficit remedied by the PEC (macrophage) infusion. It is apparent also that the alloantigens of the graft are not altered by the culture procedure in such a way that they do not serve as adequate targets for the T killer cells. As discussed elsewhere by Bach[28], allograft rejection appears to require two types of alloantigenic stimuli, denoted SD and LD. LD alloantigens have been shown to exist primarily on macrophages and B cells, whereas SD are more generally distributed on all cells. Sollinger and Bach[29] have shown that presentation of only LD alloantigens accelerated the rejection of cultured allogeneic thy-

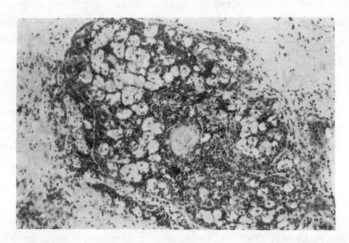

Figure 3. Human thymus cultured in 100% oxygen for 48 hours.
Large vacuolated areas are destroyed macrophages.

roid transplants.

Further manipulation in vivo or in vitro might more effi-
ciently or rapidly accomplish the elimination or inactivation of
the macrophage or other stimulator cell. Sollinger et al have
used antilymphocyte globulin and irradiation with some success
in xenogeneic transplants[10]. A very promising technique is suggested by the work of Talmage et al[30]. Culture of thyroid tissue in hyperbaric oxygen prolonged acceptance, ostensibly by
destroying macrophages (Fig. 3)

SPECIAL THYMUS EFFECT

In most cultured organ transplants, there is no effect upon
the host immune system. However, in the case of thymus transplants in nude mice, specific tolerance is produced for the alloantigens of the thymus donor[23,31]. Thus, a nude mouse (BALB/c)
transplanted with C57 Bl/6 thymus is fully tolerant of C57 Bl/6
skin or heart for periods of over one year[23,32]. The reconsti-
tuted animal retains normal allograft rejection capacity for all
other alloantigens.

This observation may be of key importance in manipulation
of the allograft rejection reaction. It is not known at the
present whether this type of specific negative adaptation can be
induced in animals with intact thymuses. If so, a clinically
important means of augmenting graft acceptance is at hand.

ACKNOWLEDGEMENTS

Supported by NIH grant AI 14354

REFERENCES

1. Jacobs, B. B., and R. A. Huseby. 1967. Successful growth of tumor allografts following culture explanation. Transplantation 5: 410.

2. Jacobs, B. B. 1974. Ovarian allograft survival. Prolongation after passage in vitro. Transplantation 18: 454.

3. Leuker, O. C., and T. R. Sharpton. 1974. Survival of ovarian allografts following maintenance in organ culture. Transplantation 18: 457.

4. Lafferty, K. J., M. A. Cooley, J. Woolnough, and K. R. Walker. 1975. Thyroid graft immunogenicity is reduced after a period in organ culture. Science 188: 259.

5. Hegre, O. D., R. J. Leonard, R. V. Schmitt, and A. Lazarow. 1976. Isotransplantation of organ cultured neonatal pancreas: reversal of alloxan diabetes in the rat. Diabetes 25: 180.

6. Starling, J. R., R. Fidler, and R. S. Corry. 1977. Prolongation of survival of rat parathyroid allografts by enhancing serum and tissue culture. Surgery 81: 668.

7. Schulte-Wissermann, H., D. Manning, and R. Hong. 1978. Transplantation of cultured thymic fragments. I. Morphologic and technical considerations. Scand. J. Immunol. 8: 387.

8. Willis, J. I. and R. L. St. Pierre. 1976. Immunological reconstitution of neonatally thymectomized rats following transplantation of thymic epithelial cells. Adv. Exp. Med. Biol. 73A: 111.

9. Jordan, R. K., D. A. Crouse, and J. J. T. Owen. 1979. Studies on the thymic microenvironment: nonlymphoid cells responsible for transferring the microenvironment. J. Reticuloendothel. Soc. 26: 373.

10. Sollinger, H. W., P. M. Burkholder, W. R. Rasmus, and F. H. Bach. 1971. Prolonged survival of xenografts after organ culture. Surgery 81: 74.

11. Wekerle, H., I. R. Cohen, and M. Feldman. 1973. Thymus reticulum cultures confer T-cell properties on spleen cells from thymus-deprived animals. Eur. J. Immunol. 3: 748.

12. Willis-Carr, J. I., H. D. Ochs, and R. J. Wedgwood. 1978. Induction of T-lymphocyte differentiation by thymic epithelial cell monolayers. Clin. Immunol. Immunopathol. 10: 315.

13. Kruisbeck, A. M., T. E. J. M. Kröse, and J. J. Zijlstra. 1977. Increase in T cell mitogen responsiveness in rat thymocytes by thymic epithelium. Eur. J. Immunol. 7: 375.

14. Pyke, K. W. and E. W. Gelfand. 1974. Morphological and functional maturation of human thymic epithelium in culture. Nature (London) 251: 421.

15. Papiernik, M., B. Nabarra, and J. F. Bach. 1975. In vitro culture of functional human thymic epithelium. Clin. Exp. Immunol. 19: 281.

16. Kukreja, S. C., P. A. Johnson, G. Ayala, E. N. Bowser and G. A. Williams. 1979. Allotransplantation of rat parathyroid glands: Effects of organ culture and transplantation into the adrenal gland. Experientia 35: 559.

17. Borzy, M. S., R. Hong, S. D. Horowitz, E. Gilbert, D. Kaufman, W. DeMendonca, V-A. Oxelius, M. Dictor, and L. Pachman. 1979. Fatal lymphoma after transplantation of cultured thymus in children with combined immunodeficiency disease. N. Engl. J. Med. 301: 565.

18. Nakagawara, G., G. Yamasaki, S. Kimura, Y. Kojima, and I. Miyazaki. 1978. Insulin-releasing activity and successful transplantation of pancreatic islets preserved by tissue culture. Surgery 83: 188.

19. Schulte-Wissermann, H., M. S. Borzy, R. Albrecht, and R. Hong. 1979. Functional relationship of macrophages and basophils to the thymus gland. Scand. J. Immunol. 9: 45.

20. Lafferty, K. J., A. Roote, G. Dart, and D. W. Talmage. 1976. Effect of organ culture on allogeneic thyroid grafts in mice. Transplantation 26: 19.

21. Pyke, K. W., H. M. Kosch, M. M. Ipp, and E. W. Gelfand. 1975. Intrathymic defect in severe combined immunodeficiency disease. N. Engl. J. Med. 293: 424.

22. Pahwa, R. N., S. G. Pahwa, and R. A. Good. 1978. T-lymphocyte differentiation in severe combined immunodeficiency: defects of the thymus. Clin. Immunol. Immunopathol. 11: 437.

23. Hong, R., H. Schulte-Wissermann, E. Jarrett-Toth, S. D. Horowitz, and D. D. Manning. 1979. Transplantation of cultured thymic fragments. II. Results in nude mice. J. Exp. Med. 149: 398.

24. Hong, R., H. Schulte-Wissermann, and S. D. Horowitz. 1979. Thymic transplantation for relief of immunodeficiency diseases. Surg. Clin. North Am. 59: 299.

25. Snell, G. D. 1957. The homograft reaction. Ann. Rev. Microbiol. 11: 439.

26. Billingham, R. E. 1971. The passenger cell concept in transplantation immunology. Cell. Immunol. 2: 1.

27. Talmage, D. W., G. Dart, J. Radovich, and K. J. Lafferty. 1976. Activation of transplant immunity: effect of donor leukocytes on thyroid allograft rejection. Science 191: 385.

28.   Bach, F. H. these proceedings.

29.   Sollinger, H. W., and F. H. Bach. 1976. Collaboration between in vivo responses to LD and SD antigens of major histocompatibility complex. Nature 259: 487.

30.   Talmage, D. W., and G. A. Dart. 1978. Effect of oxygen pressure during culture on survival of mouse thyroid allografts.
Science 200: 1066.

31.   Isaak, D. D. 1978. Fate of skin grafts from different inbred strains on nude mice bearing allogeneic thymus grafts. J.
Reticuloendothel. Soc. 23: 231.

32.   Splitter, G. A., T. C. McGuire, and W. C. Davis. 1977. The
differentiation of bone marrow cells to functional lymphocytes
following implantation of thymus grafts and thymic stroma in
nude and ATxBM mice. Cell. Immunol. 34: 93.

Organ culture of corneal tissue

Donald J.Doughman, M.D.

Department of Ophthalmology, University of Minnesota, Minneapolis, Minnesota 55455

ABSTRACT

We have been studying immunologic modification of organ cultured animal and human corneas since 1972. Guinea pig and chicken intralamellar xenografts into rabbits are modified immunologically if organ cultured at least three weeks. This may be secondary to reduction in cellularity of the donor corneas that occurs during organ culture. Human xenograft rejection was not modified regardless of organ culture duration suggesting species specificity. The data is inconclusive at this time as to whether animal allografts or human allografts are immunologically modified by organ culture storage.

INTRODUCTION

Immune modification following organ culture has been reported with a variety of rat and mice allografts[1,2,3], cultured lymphocytes[4], ovarian allografts[5,6], thyroid allografts[7] and xenografts[8], and rabbit vitreous cells[9]. In 1972 we began work in this area in conjunction with William T. Summerlin who at that time was with Robert A. Good at the University of Minnesota. Summerlin had found immune modification of skin allografts in mice[10] and humans[10,11] after six weeks in organ culture. Due to the histologic similarity and common embryologic derivation of skin and cornea, we began studies to see if there was immune modification of the organ cultured cornea. Our investigations have included experimental xenograft and allograft models as well as studies of the antigenic composition of cultured bovine corneas. In addition, we have followed human corneal transplant recipients who have received organ cultured donor corneas over the past four and one-half years in whom we have data regarding the frequency and severity of immune rejections.

ORGAN CULTURE METHOD

All organ culture procedures including preparation of globe, preparation of media, changing of media, etc. are performed utilizing sterile technique in a vertical laminar flow hood with a technician wearing a face mask, cap, gown, and sterile globes. The globes are vigorously irrigated with 50 cc sterile saline and immersed in 3% gentamicin solution for five minutes. The cornea with a 2-3 mm scleral rim is then carefully sectioned without loss of the anterior chamber. The cornea is placed epithelial side down in a sterile tissue culture Petri dish containing fresh medium (see Table for constituents of medium) and incubated for 45 minutes at 37°C. The cornea is then transferred into three separate washes of medium and dipped gently five times in each Petri dish. It is then placed epithelial side down to a fourth Petri dish, making sure medium completely covers both the scleral rim and cornea. This dish is then placed in a water jacketed tissue culture incubator at 37°C and an atmosphere of 5% CO_2, 95% filtered air, and 100% humidity. The medium is changed three times a week.

TABLE

ORGAN CULTURE MEDIA
1. Minimum essential media (Eagle's) with Earle's salts without L-glutamine (500 ml.)
2. Decomplemented calf or recipient serum (50 ml.)
3. L-glutamine (5 ml.)
4. Penicillin (100 units/ml.)
5. Gentamicin (100 µg/ml.)
6. Amphotericin B (0.25 µg/ml.)

ANIMAL STUDIES

Experimental Xenografts

Our preliminary studies indicated immune modification of chicken to rabbit intralamellar corneal xenografts after four weeks organ culture.[12] We expanded this work to include greater number of chicken xenografts as well as guinea pig and human xenograft to rabbits.[13] We found that chicken and guinea pig xenografts organ cultured at least three weeks had statistically significantly delayed rejection times compared to fresh controls. In addition, 22% of the chicken xenografts organ cultured four weeks did not reject. Human xenograft rejection was not delayed.

This indicated species specificity. Nonrejected organ cultured
xenografts as well as those xenografts with delayed rejection
times were histologically hypocellular with a decrease in or
absence of the donor epithelium. This suggested that prolonged
survival of xenografts after organ culture represented reduced
antigenicity secondary to donor hypocellularity. Recently, we
have found experimental xenografts made nonviable and hypocellular by repeated freezing and thawing or viable xenografts
with the epithelium removed prior to transplantation have
delayed rejection time similar in magnitude to organ cultured
xenografts.[14] This supports the hypothesis that organ cultured corneal xenograft modification may be related to hypocellularity. Contrary to our findings, BenEzra and Sachs could
not demonstrate immunologic modification of short term (2 to 14
days) organ cultured bovine to rabbit intralamellar xenografts.[15]

Extrapolation of results from experimental xenograft
studies to allograft immunology is not warranted according to
Silverstein since such grafts carry with them a variety of
species specific antigens which may introduce many variables
and have nothing to do with allograft immunology.[16]

Experimental Allograft

Like the experimental xenograft model, all of our experimental allografts have been done with intralamellar keratoplasties to eliminate the many non-immunologic causes of graft
failure that can occur following penetrating keratoplasty.
Since the allograft response in rabbit is weak and variable,
all our studies have involved either "second set" studies[17] or
prior sensitization of the rabbit with skin grafts from the
donor. We have unpublished data that show no evidence of immune
modification in the previously sensitized recipient. However,
second set rejection of organ cultured corneas were delayed in
some groups when compared to fresh controls. Due to variation
of results between the groups studied we do not feel conclusions
are warranted until these experiments are repeated with larger
number of experimental animals.

We have reported that three week organ cultured bovine
corneas lack a strong antigenic protein present in normal
bovine corneas.[18] Although this is due in part to loss of
epithelium during organ culture, the antigen was absent from

the stroma as well. It is likely that during organ culture loss occurs of soluble antigens known to accelerate the heterograft rejection.[19]

Effect of Autologous, Homologous or Heterologous Serum in the Organ Culture Media

Stocker[20] and Kuwahara[21] found that storing the donor cornea in recipient (autologous) serum modified the immune graft reaction. Geeraets[22] reported similar findings using homologous serum. We have found that bovine organ cultured corneas absorbed the serum protein present in the media during organ culture.[18] There seems, therefore, to be a theoretical advantage in using homologous or autologous rather than heterologous serum in the media. We tested this hypothesis in four week organ cultured chicken to rabbit intralamellar xenografts and found that although autologous and heterologous serum did delay the xenograft reaction when compared to fresh controls, homologous serum did not.[13] Comparing autologous with heterologous serum, there was no difference in delayed rejection time between the two groups. Therefore, in this model there was no immunologic advantage of autologous vs. heterologous serum.

Antigenic Modification of Organ Cultured Rabbit Conjunctival Allografts

We have unpublished data showing apparent modification of rabbit conjunctival allografts after three weeks organ culture. Since conjunctival allografts had not been previously reported we had to establish the normal clinical rejection pattern which, in our model proved to be subtle, but possible when supplemented with histology. We found 66% of the conjunctival allografts appeared to survive after three weeks organ culture. However, the cell population of these allografts was markedly reduced after organ culture. As with corneal xenografts this reduced cellularity may be playing a role in this apparent immune modification of conjunctival tissue after organ culture.

CLINICAL STUDIES

We began to use organ culture incubation as a method of long term storage for human penetrating keratoplasties in January, 1974. One hundred sixty-seven grafts have been done

of which 69.5% are clear and 30.5% have failed. The storage
duration in organ culture prior to surgery averaged 14.7 days
(range 2-37).

As of this writing, immune graft rejection accounted for
11 of 51 (22%) of the graft failures. Since the diagnosis of
immune corneal graft rejection is entirely a clinical diagnosis,
we used criteria suggested by Jones[23,24] and others[25,26,27].
An unequivocable clinical diagnosis of allograft reaction was
made when, at least ten days after transplantation, a previously
clear graft in a quiet eye rapidly developed edema with signs
of inflammation in the anterior segment including ciliary flush,
cells and flare in the anterior chamber and an endothelial
rejection line. We made a presumptive diagnosis of immune graft
rejection when all of the signs were present as stated above
but without an endothelial rejection line. If non-immune
reasons for late graft failure were present such as glaucoma,
microbial or viral infection, surgical trauma or wound
dehiscence, we did not diagnose immune rejection. In addition
to the 11 failures, 11 other grafts had rejection episodes that
were reversed with topical and systemic steroids. Most graft
reactions are said to occur during the first post-operative
year.[28] Our average duration of follow-up is now 24 months.
Polack has estimated that immune rejection of the cornea occurs
in 9%-12% of good and 40% of bad prognosis cases.[29] Based upon
our length of follow-up and the number of good and bad prognosis
cases in our series, we would have expected 27-35 immune
rejections to have occurred. Since we have diagnosed only 22,
this may mean there is some modification of the immune response
after organ culture incubation. However, without a prospective
randomized clinical study comparing organ culture storage to
another method, uncontrolled factors such as patient selection
and observer bias, not immune modification may account for these
observations.

We have replaced the fetal calf serum (heterologous) with
recipient serum (autologous) in 13 cases. All corneas remained
clear. There have been three rejection episodes in two patients
with keratoconus, all reversed with topical steroids. This data
is too small in numbers to make conclusions other than immune
rejection is not prevented using 10% autologous serum in this

system.

DISCUSSION

Our experimental animal data indicates that any effect organ culture has on corneal antigenicity is most likely due to hypocellularity of the cultured tissue. Although Ninnemann and Good could not confirm Summerlin's results in organ cultured allografts of skin[30], there seems to be abundant evidence that there is modification of immunogenicity after passage through organ culture with other cells and tissues. Lafferty has suggested that survival of thyroid allografts after in vitro culture of donor tissue is due to removal of passenger lymphocytes which play a major role of sensitization of hosts to foreign antigens of thyroid tissues.[7] Recent studies by Lacy, et. al. have confirmed this concept.[31] They performed in vitro culture of islet cells at $24^{\circ}C$ for seven days prior to transplantation in conjunction with a single injection of antiserum to lymphocytes into the diabetic recipient. This resulted in islet allograft survival of 100 days when the islets were transplanted across histocompatibility barriers. The role of passenger lymphocytes in corneal graft rejection is not known at this time.

Our studies indicate that organ culture of corneal tissue as performed in our laboratory in experiment xenografts has an effect on corneal antigenicity. However, our data regarding allograft modification in animals and humans is inconclusive at this time.

REFERENCES

1. Jacobs, B.B. 1970. Altered host-allograft relationships for mouse tumors modified by prior passage in vitro and in vivo. J. Natl. Cancer. Inst. 45: 263.
2. Jacobs, B.B. and R.A. Haughsby. 1967. Growth of tumors and allogenic hosts following organ culture explantation. Transplantation 5: 410.
3. Swaen, G.J.V. 1963. Homotransplantation of explanted tissue. Transplantation 1: 187.
4. Opelz, G. and P.I. Terasaki. 1974. Lymphocyte antigenicity loss with retention of responsiveness. Science 184: 464.
5. Jacobs, B.B. and D.E. Uphoff. 1974. Immunologic modification: A basic survival mechanism. Science 185: 582.
6. Ninnemann, J.L. and R.A. Good. 1975. Allotransplantation of murine tissue after organ culture. Fed. Proc. 34: 3645.

7. Lafferty, K.J., M.A. Cooley, J. Woolnough, and K.Z. Walker. 1975. Thyroid allograft immunogenicity is reduced after a period in organ culture. Science 188: 259.

8. Sollinger, H.W., P.M. Barkholder, W.R. Rasmus, and F.H. Bach. 1977. Prolonged survival of xenografts after organ culture. Surgery 81: 74.

9. Francois, J. and V. Victoria-Troncoso. 1973. Transplantation of vitreous cell culture. Ophthalmic Res. 4: 270.

10. Summerlin, W.T. 1973. Allogenic transplantation of organ cultures of adult skin. Clin. Immunol. Immunopathol. 1: 372.

11. Summerlin, W.T., C. Broutbar, R.B. Foanes, R. Payne, Ol Stutman, L. Hayflick, and R.A. Good. 1973. Acceptance of phenotypically differing cultured skin in man and mice. Transplant Proc. 5: 707.

12. Summerlin, W.T., G.E. Miller, M.E. Garcia, D.J. Doughman, and J.E. Harris. 1973. Transplantation of organ cultured cornea - an in vitro and in vivo study. Fed. Proc. 32: 3624.

13. Doughman, D.J., G.E. Miller, E.A. Mindrup, M.K. Schmitt, J.E. Harris, and R.A. Good. 1976. The fate of experimental organ cultured corneal xenografts. Transplantation 22: 132.

14. Doughman, D.J., L. Minaai, and E.A. Mindrup. 1979. The antigenicity of non-viable experimental corneal xenografts. Documenta Ophthalmologica 18: 263.

15. BenEzra, D. and A. Sachs. 1975. Growth and transplantation of organ cultured corneas. Invest. Ophthalmol. 14: 24.

16. Silverstein, A.M. and A.A. Khodadoust. 1973. Transplantation immunobiology of the cornea. Corneal Graft Failure. Ciba Foundation Symp. 15: 103.

17. Maumenee, E.A. 1951. The influence of donor-recipient sensitization on corneal grafts. Am. J. Ophthalmol. 34: 141.

18. Hall, J.N., G. Smolin, D.J. Doughman, H. Krasnobrod, and M.K. Schmitt. 1975. Changes in the antigenic composition of cultured bovine corneas. Invest. Ophthalmol. 14:293.

19. Leibowitz, H.M. and A.J. Luzzio. 1970. Transplantation antigens in keratoplasty. Arch. Ophthalmol. 83: 215.

20. Stocker, F.W. 1965. Preservation of donor cornea in autologous serum. Am. J. Ophthalmol. 60: 21.

21. Kuwahara, T. 1961. Studies of heterokeratoplasty. Jap. J. Ophthalmol. 5: 243.

22. Geeraets, W.J., I.R. Lederman, H. Woo, and D. Guerry. 1965. In vivo corneal graft reaction after short term storage. Am. J. Ophthalmol. 60: 28.

23. Jones, B.R. 1973. Introduction to the problems of corneal graft failure. Corneal Graft Failure. Ciba Symp. 15: 1.

24. Jones, B.R. 1973. Summing up present knowledge and problems of corneal graft failure. Corneal Graft Failure. Ciba Symp. 15: 349.

25. Polack, F.M. 1977. The corneal graft reaction. Corneal Transplantation., New York, Grune and Stratton, p. 201.

26. Khodadoust, A.A. and A.M. Silverstein. 1969. Transplantation and rejection of individual cell layers of the cornea. Invest. Ophthalmol. 8: 180.

27. Khodadoust, A.A. 1973. The allograft rejection: The leading cause of late failure of clinical corneal grafts. Corneal Graft Failure. Ciba Symp. 15: 151.

28. Fine, M. and M. Stein. 1973. The role of corneal vascularization in human corneal graft reactions. Corneal Graft Failure. Ciba Symp. 15: 193.

29. Polack, F.M. 1973. Corneal transplantation. Invest. Ophthalmol. 12: 85.
30. Ninnemann, G.L. and R.A. Good. 1974. Allogenic transplantation of organ cultures without immunosuppressants. Transplantation 8: 1.
31. Lacy, P.E., J.M. Davie, and E.H. Finke. 1979. Prolongation of islet allograft survival following in vitro Culture (24°C) and a single injection of ALS. Science 204: 312.

Modification of host responsiveness

Frank W.Fitch, M.D., Ph.D.

The Committee on Immunology and the Department of Pathology, University of Chicago, Chicago, Illinois 60637

ABSTRACT
Antibody and cell-mediated immune responses can be modulated
specifically by antigen, antibody, or anti-idiotypic (anti-receptor)
antibody acting at different stages in the complicated series of cellular
and molecular events that are initiated by immunization. Masking of
antigenic determinants by antibody can interfere with induction of immune
responses. Antigen processing can be altered by antibody to inhibit or
augment particular responses. Antibody or antigen-antibody complexes can
interact directly with particular populations of cells to modify their
reactivity; the Fc portion of the antibody molecule is required in some
instances for antibody to be suppressive. Anti-idiotypic antibody can
modulate immune responses either by reacting directly with antigen
receptors on effector B or T lymphocytes or their precursors or by
activating either helper or suppressor regulatory T lymphocytes which then
act on effector lymphocytes.

INTRODUCTION

Antigen initiates interactions among several different types of
cells having varied developmental backgrounds. In most instances, both
antibody and lymphocytes which carry out various effector functions are
produced. Regulatory lymphocytes capable of augmenting or inhibiting both
antibody and cell-mediated responses are activated at different times after
immunization. The specific reactants involved in immune responses -
antigen, specifically reactive lymphoid cells, or antibody - must
participate in those processes which result in selective modification of
immune responses. Each of these reactants has been used experimentally to
manipulate immune responses with varying degrees of success. Various
aspects of modification of immune responses have been reviewed extensively
in the past[1-9]. The effects of anti-receptor antibody on immune
responses and immunological circuits which regulate immune responses will
be considered elsewhere in this volume. This review will be concerned
mainly with the effects of passively administered antibody, either alone or
in combination with antigen.

Although experimental observations often have concentrated on one aspect of the immune response, both antibody and cell-mediated immunity usually develop after immunization. It seems likely that a given set of regulatory lymphocytes may participate in events modulating both types of responses. Passively-administered antibody acting either on antigen or regulatory cells can modulate both types of immune response. For convenience, the following discussion will consider separately the effects of passive immunization on antibody and cell-mediated immune responses, although this distinction is an artificial one.

Mechanisms of immunosuppression produced by passively administered antibody frequently have been categorized on the basis of presumed sites of action: afferent mechanisms interfere with the stimulation of antigen-reactive cells by antigen, central mechanisms directly affect immuno-competent cells or their precursors, while efferent mechanisms prevent generation of effector materials by interfering with interaction between antigen and sensitized lymphocytes or particular classes in antibodies. However, this scheme for categorizing mechanisms of immunosuppression was proposed before the complexity of cellular events of the immune response was appreciated fully. With development of better methods for studying cellular interactions, it has become evident that some examples of antibody mediated immunosuppression thought to be due to afferent or efferent blocking actually involve central mechanisms. As will be discussed below, some of the regulatory effects of antibody involve particular sub-populations of lymphocytes and may influence preferentially particular features of immune responses.

Experimental observations concerning the effects of passively administered antibody on immune responses often appear to be contra-dictory. The several immunosuppressive mechanisms need not be mutually exclusive; for a given antigen and antibody, the dominant effect of passively administered antibody may depend upon the time of administration, the relative amount, the molecular class, and the specificity of the anti-body. The affinity of antibody is an important consideration regardless of the mechanism by which it modulates the immune response since all mechanisms for specific immunoregulation by antibody involve inter-action of antibody with an antigenic determinant of some sort. Antibody of higher affinity has a greater suppressive effect on active antibody formation when given passively than does the same amount of antibody having a lower affinity[10]. The molecular class of antibody can influence the effect observed depending upon the particular mechanism of

modification that is involved. In general, IgG antibody has greater
suppressive activity than IgM antibody, and IgG subclasses may differ in
the effects that they produce[11-15].

MODIFICATION OF ANTIBODY RESPONSES BY ANTIGEN-SPECIFIC ANTIBODY

Afferent mechanisms of immunoregulation: There are relatively few
instances in which antibody seems to modulate immune responses only as a
result of its interaction with stimulating antigen. Afferent "masking" of
antigenic determinants may account for immunosuppression observed when
large amounts of antibody, in relation to the amount of antigen, are
administered passively[1,16]. This mechanism also may operate in
determinant-specific immunosuppression. In these situations, passively
administered antibody reactive with one antigenic determinant on a molecule
inhibits the active antibody response to that determinant while the
response to other determinants on the same molecule is not suppressed[17].
However, as will be discussed below, this effect is not always observed,
and passively administered antibody may modulate the response to all
determinants on a molecule or particle through mechanisms other than
antigen "masking".

Efferent mechanisms of immunoregulation: Efferent blocking by antibody
to prevent generation of effector molecules also probably occurs
infrequently. Efferent blocking of release of biologically active
materials from mast cells may occur. Circulating antibody of other immunoglobulin classes may prevent antigen from reacting with mast cell-bound IgE
and thus prevent an allergic reaction[18].

Central mechanisms of immunoregulation: Most other examples of
modulation of immune responses by passively administered antibody
(including several which superficially seem to involve afferent or efferent
mechanisms) involve direct interaction of antibody or antigen-antibody
complexes with cells. There are several different ways in which antibody
can interact with cells to modify immune responses.

Cytophilic antibody bound to non-lymphoid accessory cells or
macrophages in vitro in the absence of antigen can account for the direct
immunosuppressive effect of antibody on specific antibody responses of
spleen cells to antigen administered later[19-21]. This inhibition is
related to interaction of antibody with cells via the Fc portion of the
molecule: direct binding of intact antibody molecules has been
demonstrated, and $F(ab')_2$ fragments lacking the Fc portion of the
molecule were not immunosuppressive[19]. Some evidence suggests that this
mechanism can operate in vivo[22]. Antibody bound to macrophages may

inhibit immune responses by modifying tissue localization or cellular processing of antigen.

Alteration in antigen distribution or processing of antigen probably accounts for the augmentation of antibody response which is observed occasionally after passive immunization with IgM antibody[23-25]. This phenomenon is observed with small doses of antigen, and the magnitude of the response developed after passive immunization is not greater than that induced by "optimal" amounts of antigen. IgM antibody must be given before antigen to cause augmentation of antibody responses; given after antigen, suppression is produced[24]. Alteration in processing of antigen also may account for the well known observation that ABO incompatibility between mother and fetus diminishes the risk of Rh sensitization as well as the finding that passive immunization of individuals having O, Rh-negative erythrocytes with anti-A antibodies prevents sensitization to both A and Rh erythrocyte antigens[26]. Such a mechanism can account for inhibition of antibody response to several histocompatibility antigens produced by monoclonal antibody reactive with a single determinant[27] as well as some other situations in which augmentation or inhibition of antibody response to one set of determinants is produced by passive immunization with antibody directed toward other determinants on the same molecule[28].

Other mechanisms account for at least some of the effects of passive immunization on responses to "carrier" or "hapten" determinants on the same molecule. In most experiments evaluating the effect of passive immunization on responses to haptens, antigen has been injected with adjuvant in order to obtain appreciable antibody responses, and adjuvants may overcome, at least partially, the immunosuppressive effects of passively administered antibody[29]. In many studies, animals have been "primed" with carrier in order to increase the number of carrier-specific T cells having helper function for anti-hapten responses[30]. This may be important since secondary responses are relatively less susceptible to the inhibitory effects of passively administered antibody[1]. Given these variables, it is not surprising that apparently conflicting findings have been reported.

Passive immunization with anti-carrier antibody has been reported to produce both augmentation[31,32] and inhibition[13,14,33-36] of anti-hapten antibody responses. Generally, however, inhibition has been produced by large amounts of antibody with augmentation being observed when smaller amounts of either anti-carrier or anti-hapten antibody were given[31,37]. Although anti-carrier antibody was found to cause inhibition of antibody response to the carrier, development of carrier-specific helper T cells was unaffected[33,35]. Anti-hapten antibody usually caused suppression of active anti-hapten responses without affecting anti-carrier responses, and the apparent extent of suppression produced by anti-hapten antibody was considerably greater than that caused by anti-carrier antibody[34,38].

Several generalizations can be made about these observations. On hapten-carrier conjugates, native determinants as well as the added hapten groups can function as haptens, and several different carrier determinants may be present on a given molecule. B cells respond to hapten determinants while T cells respond to carrier determinants that may not be the same as those with which anti-carrier antibody reacts. T and B cell cooperation usually is required for antibody responses to hapten-carrier conjugates. Small amounts of anti-carrier or anti-hapten antibody may enable more effective antigen distribution and thus facilitate cooperation between T and B cells. Larger amounts of anti-hapten antibody may interfere with interaction of hapten with hapten-specific B cells but leave the response of carrier-specific T and B cells unaffected. Larger amounts of anti-carrier antibody may block carrier sites and interfere with interactions of carrier-specific helper T cells with hapten-specific and carrier-specific B cells with consequent suppression of anti-hapten and anti-carrier antibody responses. The antibody or antigen-antibody complexes could interfere with cooperative interaction between T and B cells by activating suppressor T cells which in turn inhibit helper T cell function.

Other evidence also supports the concept that the cooperation of T and B cells can be altered by passive immunization. Specific antibody added to cultures prepared with mouse spleen cells and sheep erythrocytes inhibited an active antibody response to the sheep erythrocytes. However, antibody-forming B cells or their precursors were not inactivated in this situation since the antibody-mediated suppression of specific antibody production could be reversed by addition of irradiated allogeneic cells to such cultures[39]. The irradiated allogeneic cells provided a stimulus for a mixed leukocyte reaction which can lead to production of factors capable of substituting for helper T cells in some antibody responses[40]. In this experimental system, passively administered antibody appeared to interfere with activation of helper T cells; normal antibody formation resulted if an alternative source of T cell help was provided.

Similar results were observed in other experiments in which a potent substitute for helper T cells reversed the immunosuppressive effects of low concentrations of IgG antibody while having no effect on the immun-

suppression produced by high antibody concentrations[16]. These latter
experiments provide an example of a system in which the particular
mechanism of antibody-mediated immunosuppression was dependent upon
antibody dose: inhibition of cooperative interaction between T and B cells
was caused by low concentrations of antibody while masking of antigenic
determinants was a major mechanism only at high antibody concentrations.
It is of interest that $F(ab')_2$ fragments of antibody were able to inhibit
active antibody formation only through the antigen-masking mechanism[16].

In many instances, it is not possible to distinguish whether modulation
is produced by antibody alone or by antigen-antibody complexes; antigen
stimulation is required in order to determine if responsiveness has been
altered by passive immunization, and this leads to the formation of immune
complexes. Direct suppression of cellular reactivity can be produced by
antigen-antibody complexes. Preincubation of spleen cells with mixtures of
antigen and antibody markedly and specifically suppressed the response of
spleen cells to that antigen leaving the response to another antigen
unaffected[41,42]. In this model system, incubation of cells with either
antigen or antibody alone had no effect on antibody response. Specific
inhibition was dependent upon an optimal ratio of antigen to antibody in
the complexes[44]. This effect also could be observed _in vivo_ after
injection of "subimmunogenic" amounts of antigen and antibody, and this
type of antibody-mediated unresponsiveness could be produced by amounts of
antibody undetectable in other assays[44]. Such a mechanism may account
for the phenomenon of "low zone tolerance", a situation in which injection
of an amount of antigen smaller than that required to induce antibody
formation renders an animal unresponsive to subsequent challenge with
optimal amounts of antigen[2].

Antibody secretion by activated B lymphocytes can be inhibited by
antigen-antibody complexes. Specific immune complexes have been claimed to
cause sharp reduction in the rate of secretion of antibody by lymphoid
cells[45]. This effect probably is produced by the antigen component of
the complex since exposure to antigen alone may cause a similar
effect[46]. Selective inhibition of T helper cell activity seems to be due
to cell-bound immune complexes in some model systems[47].

MODIFICATION OF CELL-MEDIATED RESPONSES BY ANTIGEN-SPECIFIC ANTIBODY

Paradoxical enhancement of tumor growth produced by active or passive
immunization is considered to be due to interference with cell-mediated
immune responses[3,4,6]. However, the complexity of the reactions which
determine the fate of tumors has led to development of other model systems

to evaluate more directly the effects of antibody on cell-mediated immunity. Passive immunization has been found to suppress at least partially the development of specific cell-mediated responses to foreign proteins[48], heterologous erythrocytes[49], and allogeneic cells[50]. The extent of suppression, although often impressive, may not be as marked as that observed for antibody formation. This may be due in part to the requirement for endogenous or exogenous adjuvants for induction of prominent cell-mediated immunity; at least for some antibody responses, adjuvants may overcome to a considerable extent inhibition produced by passive immunization[29].

Distinctions have been made between mechanisms involving antibody effects on recognition and effector phases of cell-mediated immunity. "Masking" of antigenic determinants by passively administered antibody can account for inhibition of both proliferative[51-54] and cytolytic responses[55,56]. It is also possible for antibody directed toward Ia antigens expressed on macrophages to inhibit interaction between macrophages and T cells and thus prevent helper T cell activation[57,58]. Antibody also can interfere with the interaction between sensitized effector lymphocytes and antigen. Antibody directed toward histocompatibility antigens on target cells could effectively inhibit cell-mediated cytotoxicity in the ^{51}Cr-release assay in vitro[59]. However, all antigens must be blocked since antibody directed against one set of antigens expressed on target cells is unable to prevent the lytic effect of T lymphocytes reactive with another set of antigens present on the same target cells[60]. In any case, this mechanism is unlikely to be important in preventing target cell injury in vivo since interaction of antibody with target cell antigens would favor opsonization or complement activation with subsequent destruction of the target cell. A least some of the "serum blocking factors" capable of inhibiting T cell-mediated cytotoxicity in animals bearing tumors or long-term renal allografts consist of antigen-antibody complexes[61]. However, it should be noted that such blocking factors may inhibit lymphocyte activity reflected in the microcytotoxicity test[62] but not that detected in the ^{51}Cr-release assay[63].

There are a number of situations in which supression of cell-mediated immune responses by passively administered antibody cannot be explained by simple blocking of recognition or effector phases of the response. For example, inhibition of an anti-allogeneic cytolytic cell response against trinitrophenyl-complexed allogeneic stimulator cells by anti-trinitrophenyl antibody is dependent upon the presence of the Fc portion of the antibody molecule[64] while the Fc portion is not required for suppression of the response of unmodified allogeneic cells by alloantibody[57]. Dose-response relationships indicate that $F(ab')_2$ antibody seppresses cell-mediated responses by a mechanism different than that by which IgG antibody causes inhibition, but this mechanism has not been characterized[64].

Allograft enhancement is another example of antibody-induced modulation of cell-mediated responses by mechanisms not yet understood. Treatment of recipient rats with donor antigen and anti-donor antibody leads to the indefinite survival of renal or cardiac allografts[65]. Although production of anti-idiotypic antibody is induced by this procedure, such antibody cannot be detected beyond the early post-transplant period[66]. Anti-idiotypic antibodies may play a role in the induction of allograft enhancement, but they seem not to account for all of the findings. Reactivity of lymphoid cells from long-term allograft recipients toward graft antigens is unimpaired when tested in vitro[67]. This observation is not consistent with the suggestion that passive immunization leads to opsonization of specific antigen-reactive cells[68]. The normal reactivity of cells from long-term recipients also seems to exclude a role for suppressor T cells which seem to be responsible for suppression of skin graft rejection in some model systems[69]. It may be that several mechanisms operate sequentially in renal allograft enhancement. In any case, this phenomenon remains an enigma.

Regardless of the immunoregulatory processes that are active, it is possible to achieve renal allograft enhancement using antibodies directed against a single determinant present on graft antigen. Homogeneous, monoclonal antibodies reactive with graft antigens have been obtained by fusing spleen cells from rats immunized against donor antigens with mouse myeloma cells[27]. Several antibodies of different molecular class and having different patterns of antibody specificity have been obtained. Some but not all of these monoclonal antibodies were able to suppress antibody formation in vivo and, when given with antigen, were able to induce allograft enhancement as effectively as whole alloimmune serum[27].

MODIFICATION OF IMMUNE RESPONSES BY ANTI-IDIOTYPIC ANTIBODY

Antibody, especially in the form of antigen-antibody complexes, can function as immunogen for induction of anti-idiotypic antibody[70]. There are several mechanisms by which anti-idiotypic antibody can modulate immune responses. These effects will be considered extensively elsewhere in this volume. It is sufficient here to point out that anti-idiotypic antibody can modify immune responses by blocking antigen receptors of B lymphocytes or by activating helper or suppressor T cells, effects that are similar operationally to those produced by passively administered antibody. Anti-idiotypic antibody may appear "spontaneously" during the course of hyperimmunization, probably induced by antigen-antibody complexes which form after repeated antigen injection[71-73]. Thus, unrecognized anti-idiotypic antibodies may be present in antibody preparations that are used for passive immunization and may account for some of the effects observed.

GENERAL COMMENTS

Indeed, it seems reasonable to follow the suggestion made several years ago by Schwarz[74] that "All parties in the controversy that exists on the immunoregulatory effects of antibody should be declared correct". Several distinct regulatory mechanisms have been documented, and the dominant process (or processes) will depend upon the particular set of circumstances. Antibody can "mask" antigen to prevent recognition by antigen-reactive cells or to block effector mechanisms. However, antibody or antigen-antibody complexes also can react with effector B and T lymphocytes and probably with helper and suppressor T cells as well . The final effect produced will depend on the amounts of antigen and antibody given and the number and proportion of the various lymphocyte sub-populations. The sequence of exposure of these cells to antigen and antibody may determine which set of regulatory events become dominant[75].

Passive immunization has been used clinically with spectacular success to prevent erythroblastosis fetalis[76]. The potential for therapuetic application methods for specific modification of host immune responses is great. However, the responses should be characterized sufficiently to permit the use of antibody or anti-idiotypic antibody to intervene at the appropriate stage of the response to achieve the desired modification while avoiding the activation of other, perhaps harmful reactions.

REFERENCES

1. Uhr, J.W., and G. Moller. 1968. Regulatory effect of antibody on the immune response. Adv. Immunol. 8: 81.
2. Dresser, D.W., and N.A. Mitchison. 1968. The mechanism of immunological paralysis. Adv. Immunol. 8: 129.
3. Kaliss, N. 1969. Immunological enhancement. Int. Rev. Exp. Path. 8: 241.
4. Voisin, G.A. 1971. Immunological facilitation, a broadening of the concept of the enhancement phenomenon. Prog. Allergy 15: 328.
5. Feldmann, M., and G.J.V. Nossal. 1972. Tolerance, enhancement, and the regulation of interactions between T-cells, B-cells, and marcrophages. Transplant. Rev. 13: 3.
6. Feldman, J.D. 1972. Immunological enhancement: a study of blocking antibodies. Adv. Immunol. 15: 167.
7. Weigle, W.O. 1973. Immunological unresponsiveness. Adv. Immunol. 16: 61.

8. Gershon, R.R. 1974. T-cell control of antibody production. Contemp. Topics Immunol. 3: 1.

9. Fitch, F.W. 1975. Selective suppression of immune responses: Regulation of antibody formation and cell-mediated immunity by antibody. Prog. Allergy. 19: 195.

10.Walker, J.G., and G.W. Siskind. 1968. Studies on the control of antibody synthesis. Effect of antibody affinity upon its ability to suppress antibody formation. Immunology 14: 21.

11. Murgita, R.A., and S.I. Vas. 1972. Specific antibody-mediated effect on the immune response. Suppressing and augmentation of the primary immune response in mice by different classes of antibodies. Immunology 22: 319.

12. Fuller, T.C., and H.J. Winn. 1973. Immunochemical and biological characterization of alloantibody active in immunological enhancement. Transplant. Proc. 5: 585.

13.Vuagnat, P., T. Neveu, and G.A. Voisin. 1973. Immunodeviation by passive antibody, an expression of selective immunodepression. I. Action of guinea pig IgG1 and IgG2 anti-hapten antibodies. Eur. J. Immunol. 3: 90.

14. Vuagnat, P., T. Neveu, and G.A. Voisin. 1973. Immunodeviation by passive antibody, an expression of selective immunodepression. II. Action of guinea pig IgG1 and IgG2 anti-carrier antibodies. J. Exp. Med. 137: 265.

15. Rubinstein, P., F. Decary, and E. W. Streun. 1974. Quantitative studies on tumor enhancement in mice. I. Enhancement of Sarcoma I induced by IgM, IgG1 and IgG2. J. Exp. Med. 140: 591.

16. Hoffmann, M.K., and J.W. Kappler. 1978. Two distinct mechanisms of immune suppression by antibody. Nature 272: 64.

17. Cerottini, J.-C., P.J. McConahey, and F.J. Dixon. 1969. Specificity of the immunosuppression caused by passive administration of antibody. J. Immunol. 103: 268.

18. Levy, D.A., L.M. Lichtenstein, E.O. Goldstein, and K. Ishizaka. 1971. Immunologic and cellular changes accompanying the therapy of pollen allergy. J. Clin. Invest. 50: 360.

19. Abrahams, S, R.A. Phillips, and R.G. Miller. 1973. Inhibition of the immune response by 7S antibody. Mechanism and site of action. J. Exp. Med. 137: 870.

20. Pierce, C.W. 1969. Immune response in vitro. II. Suppression of the immune response in vitro by specific antibody. J. Exp. Med. 130: 365.

21. Ptak, W., and J. Pryjma. 1971. Cytophilic antibody and the regulation of the immune response. Eur. J. Immunol. 1: 408.

22. Rowley, D.A., and F.W. Fitch. 1964. Homeostasis of antibody formation in the adult rat. J. Exp. Med. 120: 987.

23. Henry, C., and N.K. Jerne. 1968. Competition of 19S and 7S antigen receptors in the regulation of the primary immune response. J. Exp. Med. 128: 133.

24. Wason, W.M. 1973. Regulation of the immune response with antigen specific IgM antibody: a dual role. J. Immunol. 110: 1245.

25. Dennert, G. 1971. The mechanism of antibody-induced stimulation and inhibition of the immune response. J. Immunol. 106: 951.

26. Stern, K., H.S. Goodman, and M. Berger. 1961. Experimental isoimmunization to hemoantigens in man. J. Immunol. 87: 189.

27. McKearn, T.J., F.W. Fitch, D.E. Smilek, M. Sarmiento, and F.P. Stuart. 1979. Properties of rat anti-MHC antibodies produced by cloned rat-mouse hybridomas. Immunol. Rev. 47: 91.

28. Henney, C.S., and K. Ishizaka. 1970. Studies on the immunogenicity of antigen-antibody precipitates. II. The suppressive effect of anti-carrier and anti-hapten antibodies on the immunogenicity of dinitrophenylated human G globulin. J. Immunol. 104: 1540.

29. Rowley, D.A., F.W. Fitch, M.A. Axelrad, and C.W. Pierce. 1969. The immune response suppressed by specific antibody. Immunol. 16: 549.

30. Katz, D.H., W.E. Paul, E.A. Goidl, and B. Benacerraf. 1970. Carrier functions in anti-hapten immune responses I. Enhancement of primary and secondary anti-hapten antibody responses by carrier preimmunization. J. Exp. Med. 132: 261.

31. Pincus, C., G. Miller, and V. Nussenzweig. 1973. Enhancement of an anti-hapten response by an antiserum to the carrier protein. J. Immunol. 110: 301.

32. Terres, G., G.S. Habicht, and R.D. Stoner. 1974. Carrier-specific enhancement of the immune response using antigen-antibody complexes. J. Immunol. 112: 804.

33. Kappler, J.W., M. Hoffmann, and R.W. Dutton. 1971. Regulation of the immune response. I. Differential effect of passively administered antibody on the thymus-derived and bone marrow-derived lymphocytes. J. Exp. Med. 134: 577.

34. Hamaoka, T., K. Takatsu, and M. Kitagawa. 1973. Antibody production in mice. V. The suppressive effect oif anti-carrier antibodies on cellular cooperation in the induction of secondary anti-hapten antibody responses. Immunology 24: 409.

35. Hoffman, M.K., J.W. Kappler, J.A. Hirst, and H.F. Oettgen. 1974. Regulation of the immune response. V. Antibody-mediated inhibition of T and B cell cooperation in the in vitro response to red cell antigens. Eur. J. Immunol. 4: 282.

36. Takatsu, K., T. Hamaoka, and M. Kitagawa. 1974. Antibody production in mice. VI. Effect of anti-carrier antibody on cellular cooperation in the primary anti-hapten antibody response. Immunology 26: 233.

37. Haughton, G, and O. Makela. 1973. Suppression or augmentation of the anti-hapten response in mice by antibodies of different specificities. J. Exp. Med. 138: 103.

38. Hamaoka, T., T. Takatsu, and M. Kitagawa. 1971. Antibody production in mice. IV. The suppressive effect of anti-hapten and anti-carrier antibodies on the recognition of hapten-carrier conjugates in the secondary response. Immunology 21: 259.

39. Lees, R.K. and N.R. StC. Sinclair. 1975. Regulation of the immune response. IX. Resistance to antibody mediated immunsuppression induced by the presence of the allogeneic effect. Cell. Immunol. 17: 525.

40. Armerding, D., and D.H. Katz. 1974. Activation of T and B lymphocytes in vitro. II. Biological and biochemical properties of allogeneic effect factor (AEF) active in triggering of specific B lymphocytes. J. Exp. Med. 140: 19.

41. Feldmann, M., and E. Diener. 1970. Antibody-mediated suppression of the immune response in vitro. I. Evidence for a central effect. J. Exp. Med. 131: 247.

42. Oberbarnscheidt, J., and E. Kolsch. 1978. Direct blockade of antigen-reactive B lymphocytes by immune complexes. An "off" signal for precursors of IgM producing cells provided by the linkage of antigen-and Fc receptors. Immunology 35: 151.

43. Diener, E., and M. Feldmann. 1970. Antibody-mediated suppression of the immune response in vitro. II. A new approach to the phenomenon of immunological tolerance. J. Exp. Med. 132: 31.

44. Feldmann, M., and E. Diener. 1971. Antibody-mediated suppression of the immune response in vitro. III. Low zone tolerance in vitro. Immunology 21: 387.

45. Nossal, G.J.V. and B.L. Pike. 1974. Immunological tolerance: mechanisms and potential therapeutic applications. In: Katz, D.A. and B. Enacerraf, ed. New York, Academic Press.

46. Schrader, J.W., and G.J.V. Nossal. 1974. Effector cell blockade. A New mechanism of immune hyporeactivity induced by multivalent antigens. J. Exp. Med. 139: 1582.

47. Kontiainen, S. and N.A. Mitchison. 1975. Blocking antigen-antibody complexes on the T-lymphocyte surface identified with defined protein antigens. I. Lymphocyte activation during in vitro incubation before adaptive transfer. Immunology 28: 523.

48. Crowle, A.J., K. Yonemasu, C.C. Hu, and Y. Fujita. 1974. Characterization of contrasensitizing antibodies. Cell. Immunol. 11: 272.

49. Axelrad, M.H. Suppression of delayed hypersensitivity by antigen and antibody. Is a common precursor cell responsible for both delayed hypersensitivity and antibody formation? Immunology 15: 159.

50. Brunner, K.T., J. Mauel, and R. Schindler. 1967. Inhibitory effect of isoantibody on in vivo sensitization and on the in vitro cytotoxic action of immune lymphocytes. Nature, Lond. 213: 1246.

51. Abbasi, K,, H. Festenstein, W. Verbi, and I.M. Roitt. 1974. Dissociation of lymphocyte activating determinants from recognition sites in mouse MLR. Nature, Lond. 251: 227.

52. Gatti, R.A., E.A.J. Svedmyr, and H. Wigzell. 1974. Characterization of a serum inhibitor of MLC reactions. II. Molecular structure and dissociation of inhibition against responder and stimulator function. Cell. Immunol. 11: 466.

53. Schwartz, R.H., C.G. Fathman, and D.H. Sachs. 1976. Inhibition of stimulation of murine mixed lymphocyte cultures with an alloantiserum directed against a shared Ia determinant. J. Immunol. 116: 929.

54 Thomas, D.W., U. Yamashita, and E. Shevach. 1977. Nature of the antigenic complex recognized by T lymphocytes. IV. Inhibition of antigen-specific T cell proliferation by antibodies to stimulator macrophage Ia antigens. J. Immunol. 119: 223.

55. Lemonnier, F, S.J. Burakoff, M. Mescher, M.E. Dorf, and B. Benacerraf. 1978. Inhibition of the induction of cytolytic T lymphocytes with alloantisera directed against H-2K and H-2D gene products. J. Immunol. 120: 1717.

56. Sinclair, N.R. StC., R.K. Lees, G. Fagan, and A. Birnbaum. 1975. Regulation of the immune response. VIII. Characteristics of antibody-mediated suppression of an in vitro cell-mediated immune response. Cell. Immunol. 16: 330.

57. Pierce, C.W., J.A. Kapp, S.M. Solliday, M.E. Dorf, and B. Benacerraf. 1974. Immune responses in vitro. XI. Suppression of primary IgM and IgG plaque-forming cell responses in vitro by alloantisera against leukocyte alloantigens. J. Exp. Med. 140: 921.

58. Frelinger, J.A., J.E. Niederhuber, and D.C. Shreffler. 1975. Inhibition of immune responses in vitro by specific antisera to Ia antigens. Science. 118: 268.

59. Brunner, K.T., J. Mauel, J.-C. Cerottini, and B. Chapuis. 1968. Quantitative assay of the lytic action of immune lymphoid cells on ^{51}Cr-labelled allogeneic target cells in vitro; inhibition by isoantibody and by drugs. Immunology 14: 181.

60. Cerottini, J.-C., and K.T. Brunner. 1974. Cell-mediated cytotoxicity, allograft rejection and tumor immunity. Adv. Immunol. 18: 67.

61. Hellstrom, K.E., and I. Hellstrom. 1974. Lymphocyte-mediated cytotoxicity and blocking serum activity to tumor antigens. Adv. Immunol. 18: 209.

62. Stuart, F.P., F.W. Fitch, D.A. Rowley, J.L. Biesecker, K.E. Hellstrom, and I. Hellstrom. 1971. Presence of both cell-mediated immunity and serum-blocking factors in rat renal allografts 'enhanced' by passive immunization. Transplantation 12: 331.

63. Biesecker, J.L., F.W. Fitch, D.A. Rowley, D. Scollard, and F.P. Stuart. 1973. Cellular and humoral immunity after allogeneic transplantation in the rat. II. Comparison of a ^{51}Cr relase assay and modified microcytotoxicity assay for detection of cellular immunity and blocking serum factors. Transplantation 16: 421.

64. Sinclair, N.R. StC., and F.Y. Law. 1979. Antibody-mediated immunosuppression of a cytotoxic cell response not involving a simple antigen-masking mechanism. J. Immunol. 123: 1439.

65. Stuart, F.P., T.J. McKearn, A.Weiss, and F.W. Fitch. 1979. Suppression of rat renal allograft rejection by antigen and antibody. Immunol. Rev. 49: (in press).

66. Stuart, F.P., D.M. Scollard, T.J. McKearn, and F.W. Fitch. 1976. Cellular and humoral immunity after allogeneic transplantation in the rat. V. Appearance of anti-idiotypic antibody and its relationship to cellular immunity after treatment with donor spleen cells and alloantibody. Transplantation 22: 455.

67. Weiss, A., F.P. Stuart, and F.W. Fitch. 1978. Immune reactivity of cells from long term rat renal allograft survivors. Transplantation 26: 346.

68. Hutchinson, I.V., and H. Zola. 1977. Antigen reactive cell opsonization (ARCO). A mechanism of immunological enhancement. Transplantation 23: 464.

69. Dorsch, S., and B. Roser. 1977. Recirculating, suppressor T cells in transplantation tolerance. J. Exp. Med. 145: 1144.

70. Eichmann, K. 1978. Expression and function of idiotypes on lymphocytes. Adv. Immunol. 26: 195.

71. McKearn, T.J., F.P. Stuart, and F.W. Fitch. 1974. Anti-idiotypic antibody in rat transplantation immunity. I. Production of anti-idiotypic antibody in animals repeatedly immunized with alloantigens. J. Immunol. 113: 1876.

72. Rodkey, L.S. 1974. Studies of idiotypic antibodies. Production and characterization of autoantiidiotypic antisera. J. Exp. Med. 139: 712.

73. Kluskens, L., and H. Kohler. 1974. Regulation of immune response by autogenous antibody against receptor. Proc. Natl. Acad. Sci. USA. 71: 5083.

74. Schwartz, R.S. 1971. Immunoregulation by antibody. Prog. Immunol. 1: 1081.

75. Rowley, D.A., H. Kohler, H. Schreiber, S.T. Kaye, and I. Lorbach. 1976. Suppression by autogenous complementary idiotypes: the priority of the first response. J. Exp. Med. 144: 946.

76. Freda, V.J. J.G. Gorman, W. Pollack, and E. Bowe. 1975. Prevention of Rh hemolytic disease - ten years' clinical experience with Rh immune globulin. N. Eng. J. Med. 292: 1014.

A note on T cell receptors and anti-receptor immunity

H.Binz*, H.Frischknecht* and H.Wigzell**

*Division of Experimental Microbiology, Institute for Medical Microbiology, University of Zurich, Switzerland, and **Institute of Immunology, Box 582, BMC, S-751 23 Uppsala, Sweden

ABSTRACT

Purified T cell receptors have been analyzed as to their biochemical and serological features as they constitute the prime targets for anti-receptor regulation in transplantation system. Heterogeneity at the anti-MHC receptor level is observed at two levels: with regard to which allo-MHC molecules are being recognized and b) with regard to detectable, seemingly inducible anti-self MHC reactivity of at least some allo-MHC reactive receptors. Conditions for successful anti-receptor immunizations in the allo-MHC systems are discussed in brief as well as the need for improvments to achieve a more regular and frequent suppression in the individual animals.

INTRODUCTION

Anti-receptor immunity in the auto-anti-idiotypic sense has been proven to be a reality by several workers (initially shown by Rodkey[1]) and can involve both B and T lymphocytes[2]. The consequences of such auto-anti-idiotypic reactions seem to be as varying as the immune response itself and stimulatory as well as inhibitory consequences with regard to the idiotype-positive lymphocytes have been recorded[3,4]. In the transplantation immune systems it has by now been found possible by several workers to induce such auto-anti-idiotypic immune reactions leading in several instances to reduction or sometimes close to complete elimination of a select immune reactivity towards certain major histocompatibility antigens[2,5,6]. It is, however, quite clear that the average frequency of success is still much too low to allow the introduction of the present procedures into the clinical situation of a "normal" allogeneic graft such as a kidney transplant[7]. Still, the results obtained so far have been of importance both from theoretical as well as possible practical considerations.

In the present article we will discuss in brief the present situation with regard to the fine antigen-binding features and biochemistry of the T cell receptors with specificity for allogeneic transplantation antigens as studied using anti-receptor antibodies as well as direct binding measurements to various "target" antigens. This we do as we deem it essential to concentrate at T cell receptors as prime targets in attempted immune regulations of transplantation immunity and knowledge of the target is required for efficient control of its function(s). We do also include the present status as to our knowledge when it is or is not possible to induce immune suppression in the histocompatibility systems using anti-receptors immunizations.

Biochemistry of T cell receptors with specificity for allo-MHC antigens

We have previously presented several articles dealing with the biochemical features of T cell derived molecules being derived from rat T lymphocytes with specificity for AgB molecules of another rat strain[8]. These molecules have always been otained in a "pure" form using as immunosorbants anti-idiotypic antibodies, frequently of auto-anti-idiotypic nature. It is thus clear that our sampling procedures for obtaining such T cell receptors may suffer from inherent experimental complications in relation to receptors purified by other means. Table I presents our present understanding of these receptor molecules as to biochemical features. In the rat we have regularly obtained a sizeable fraction of these molecules in the form of dimers of two similarly sized polypeptide chains making up a molecule of close to 150 K daltons. We have been unable to separate the two chains from each other, that is we believe they are probably identical subunits. The chain in a single form can still effectuate antigen binding as well as expressing idiotypic determinant. We have also regularly found that the large chain is quite susceptible to proteolysis, yielding fragments around 50 K and 35 K daltons in size. The possibility, however, does exist that such groups of molecules as defined by size may also be released in such a form from certain T lymphocytes. A confusing issue has been the ability of the T cell-derived material to bind to protein A from Staphylococcus aureus. Using protein A-Sepharose

Table I. Biochemical features of T cell receptors with anti-MHC specificity
as defined by antigen-binding or idiotypes

Size: When isolated from T cell membranes of normal or immune T cells using
anti-idiotypic antibodies using non-reducing conditions peaks around 150.000
and 70.000 daltons dominate. The 150.000 sized molecules will turn into
70.000 upon reduction. The 70.000 sized molecules tend to sponteneously
degrade into 50.000 and 35.000 daltons molecules but attempts to prove the
70.000 molecules to be two chain structures have failed. Similar 150.000
and 70.000 molecules can be isolated from serum but are then frequently
contaminated with molecules yielding 50.000 and 25.000 sized chains. It is
possible that these molecules are from B cells. The 70.000 chain molecules
yield clearcut fragments using papain around 50K, 44K, 35K, 31K, 27K, 21K
and 15K daltons whereas pepsin produced partial fragmentations yielding
44K, 26K and 24K dalton molecules.

Antigen-binding and idiotypes: The 150K, 70K and the 50K and 35K sized
molecules do all express antigen-binding and idiotypes. The other fragments
are unknown.

Carbohydrates: Galactose oxidase-sodium borohydride techniques fail to
label the T cell molecules. 19 lectin columns covering most sugar specificities known failed to bind the soluble T cell molecules. Limited attempts
to label using tritiated sugars have also failed.

Protein A binding: Highly coupled protein A-CL-Sepharose from Pharmacia
is binding the T cell 70.000 chains whereas several protein A CNBR Sepharose
batches made in the laboratory have failed to do so.

from Pharmacia we now normally find significant binding, a
feature not encountered when using protein A-Sepharose with
somewhat lower conjugation ratios[8]. However, this does not
necessarily indicate any striking similarities between the T
cell derived polypeptides and IgG as both IgM, IgA and IgE
molecuels can be found to bind to protein A under certain conditions. From our earlier studies we know that the genes coding
for the rat T cell chain are linked to the heavy chain Ig genes
[9]. Light chains of conventional type are always lacking in our
preparations of T cell receptors. Another point of importance
is that significant amounts of carbohydrates as studied using
some 20 different lectins, internal labelling procedures with
tritiated sugars as well as sugar oxidizing enzymes have all

failed to prove the existence of such molecules on the polypeptide chains. Do also note that the degradation patterns of
the IgT chain is quite distinct using various proteolytic enzymes under controlled in vitro conditions. In all, the receptors isolated from rat T cells are at least in part clearly
distinct from other immunoglobulin molecule classes known to be
produced by B lymphocytes. In many ways the molecules seem to
most closely resemble yet be distinct from the early IgM molecules that are produced by s.c. pre-B lymphocytes[10]. Whether
this means that the T cell receptor molecules represents a
phylogenetically older branch of the immunoglobulin tree as
presented by B cells remains, however, a speculation.

Fine antigen-binding specificity of T cell receptors with
specificity for MHC determinants

Single chain molecules of T cell origin can bind quite well
to the relevant antigen[8]. In the case of the allogeneic MHC
antigens the actual determinants are not known but it is a fair
assumption from available serological and biochemical data that
the MHC antigens of the same locus group within the species
are very similar but with yet distinct unique variations making
them function like histocompatibility antigens. We have made
some attempts to analyze the fine antigen-binding ability of
isolated T cell receptors for single MHC polypeptide chains
in comparison to what is being "seen" by B cell receptors
(= IgG alloantibodies) and what is being bound to the actual
immunocompetent T lymphocyte as such. Some of these results
have been published[11,12]. In table 2 we can show that T cell
receptors in isolated form can express the expected strong and
selective affinity for some of the relevant allo-MHC chains
(in this system one group of receptors reacted with the heavy
AgG (=H-2 or HLA-ABC-like) chain, whereas another group of
molecules reacted with the heavy Ia chain). We consider it
noteworthy that the very same binding pattern was observed
when studying the binding of labelled material from stimulator
cells to responder T cells in MLC:s. Why beta$_2$ microglobulin
or light Ia chains failed to bind under the latter conditions
for the necessary time period is unknown but thoughtprovoking.
The most striking observation was, however, that significant
although weak binding was noted for the heavy "self" Ia poly-

Table 2. <u>Fine antigen-binding ability of T cell receptors for allo-MHC versus self-MHC polypeptide chains. An analysis at the molecular and cellular level</u>

A. <u>Molecular level</u>

1. Lewis-anti-DA T cell receptors purified from normal Lewis serum using auto-anti-Lewis-anti-DA idiotypic immunosorbents were coupled to Sepharose. Such columns did bind internally labelled single MHC polypeptide chains of the following types: DA heavy chain of AgB (44K) and heavy Ia of DA (34K) but not the light Ia chain of DA (27K); the bound chains were strongly bound. The heavy Ia of Lewis (self) was weakly bound = retarded. Other Lewis MHC chains did not show detectable retardation nor did MHC chains from BN rats do display any specific binding. Control IgG Lewis-anti-DA immunosorbents did bind strongly all three groups of DA MHC chains whilst failing to display any detectable binding to Lewis or BN MHC chains.

B. <u>Cellular level</u>

1. Lewis-anti-DA MLC T blasts were incubated with internally labelled DA, BN or Lewis spleen cells for some hours followed by purifications (gradients plus selective lysis of stimulator cells) to get pure T blasts. Such cells were lysed and the bound material analyzed on SDS-PAGE. Heavy AgG and heavy Ia chain molecules were found bound when using DA stimulator cells but no $beta_2$ microglobulin or light chain Ia molecules. Lewis or BN stimulator cells failed to provide MHC molecules with strong binding properties for the Lewis-anti-DA MLC T blasts.

<u>Conclusion</u>: Looks like two kinds of T cells can be identified by these binding procedures: one with specificity for the AgB chains as such and one with specificity for heavy Ia chain alloantigenic determinants (and self unique determinants).

---

peptide chains but not for 3rd party heavy Ia chains. We interpret this to in fact prove that the very same receptors that are involved in allo-MHC reactions can also participate in antiself MHC restricted responses. In some preliminary experiments we have suggestive further evidence that this reactivity towards "self" MHC indeed is opportune, that is placing the V_H gene coding for this particular T cell associated idiotype on another MHC background will now make this group of T cell receptors start to display selective weak affinity for this new "self" MHC instead of the previous self-MHC molecules. One may wonder whether this may not cause selective ablation of "good" anti-self immunity in parallel to the "bad" anti-allo-MHC reactivity when attempting auto-anti-receptor immunity? The practical results so far have failed to indicate any increased susceptibility to disease in such "tolerized" animals. Also, in practive they may rather be expected to behave like F_1 hybrids between the true genotype and the "tolerized" donor type. This has in fact never been studied (if other expected T cell associated immune reactivities associated with F_1 hybrid combinations of conventional type also will occur in auto-anti-idiotypic immunity generated "F_1:s").

Conditions under which efficient anti-receptor immunity in the allo-MHC system has been observed

Anti-receptor immunity of auto-anti-idiotypic nature causing close to complete tolerance (but very seldom exceeding the 80 % reduction level) has been observed by us in several species (mice, rats or guinea pigs) under proper conditions[8]. Similar auto-anti-idiotypic reactions have also been reported in chimpanzees[13] and baboons[6]. Many individual animals undergoing attempted anti-receptor immunization protocols fail, however, to become depressed to any significant degree. In table 3 we present the conditions under which we have or have not been able to induce significant specific immune suppression via anti-receptor immunity of a select nature. Note that they may not always be of a depressing nature but can under certain conditions be found to function like allo-MHC antigens in the stimulatory sense[4]. Adjuvanticity has also been a true problem in the autologous systems but here progress with regard to possibly "acceptable" adjuvants for potential human use has now taken place. Complexity as to receptor specificities in the various subpopulations of T lymphocytes have been noted corresponding well with expectation but obviously putting greater demands of a very diversified anti-receptor response if a relatively significant selective suppression of the anti-allo-MHC response would be expected to become induced. It is still quite clear, however, that the relative success rates as to achieve more than 75 % supression of specific nature as to T cell mediated anti-MHC reactions must

Table 3. __Conditions required for successful anti-receptor immunization__
__in the anti-allo-MHC system__

Adjuvants: In case of auto-anti-receptor immunity we have only been able
to induce this with the help of adjuvants. Two types of adjuvants have
functioned: Freund's complete adjuvant and muramyl dipeptide variants.
Adjuvants which have failed to function include Freund's incomplete adjuvant, alum precipitation and Hemophilus pertussis bacteria. Successful
anti-receptor immunization = reduction in immune responsiveness according
to our definition. It is possible to achieve auto-anti-idiotypic antibody
production using antigen-antibody complexes but in the allo-MHC system this
is frequently parallelled with immunity.

T cells better than B cells: The most efficient and simplest way of obtaining
anti-T receptor immunity has been to use antigen-specific T blasts purified
via MLC plus 1-g sedimentation in adjuvants. Idiotypic alloantibodies can
be used but here we have found heavy chains better than intact IgG molecules with regard to induction of anti-T reactive anti-receptor antibodies.
Purified B cells as such have never functioned as inducers of anti-receptor
immunity in the allo-MHC systems.

Normal versus immune conditions: It is significantly more difficult to
induce anti-receptor immunity leading to suppression in an already immune
individual. Here, only partial reduction in specific reactivity has been
achieved using autologous MLC T blasts as immunogen.

Quantity of receptors: We have so far found no exception to the rule than
within the limits used the more T cells used as auto-immunogen the greater
the likelihood for obtaining specific anti-receptor immunity.

be improved further to make the approach an attractive one for
clinical trials.

ACKNOWLEDGEMENTS

This work was supported by the Swedish Cancer Society and
by the Swiss National Science Foundation grant 3.668-76 and the
Swiss Cancer Society grant 135-AK-79.

REFERENCES

1.   Rodkey, L.L. 1974. Studies on idiotypic antibodies. Production and characterization of auto-anti-idiotypic antisera.
J.Immunol. 139: 712.
2.   Binz, H., and H. Wigzell. 1977. Idiotypic alloantigen-reactive
T lymphocyte receptors and their use to induce specific transplantation tolerance. Progr.Allerg. 23: 154.
3.   Eichmann, K., and K. Rajewsky. 1975. Induction of T and B
cell immunity by anti-idiotypic antibody. Eur.J.Immunol. 5: 661.

4. Frischknecht, H., Binz, H., and H. Wigzell. 1978. Induction of specific transplantation immune reactions using anti-idiotypic antibodies. J.Exp.Med. 147: 500.

5. Andersson, L.C., Aguet, M., Wight, E., Andersson, R., Binz, H., and H. Wigzell. 1977. Induction of specific unresponsiveness using purified MLC-activated T lymphoblasts as auto-immunogen. I. Demonstration of general validity as to species and histocompatibility barriers. J.Exp.Med. 146: 1124.

6. Myburgh, J.A., and J.A. Smit. 1979. Autoantiidiotypic immunization and transplantation in the primate. Transplant.Proc. 11: 923.

8. Binz, H., and H. Wigzell. 1976. Shared idiotypic determinants on B and T lymphocytes reactive against the same antigenic determinants. V. Biochemical and serological characteristics of naturally occurring, soluble antigen-binding T-lymphocyte derived molecules. Scand.J.Immunol. 5: 559.

9. Binz. H., Wigzell, H., and H. Bazin. 1976. Inheritance of T cell idiotypic receptors specific for transplantation antigens is linked to the genes coding for heavy chains of immunoglobulins. Nature 264: 778.

10. Burrows, P.D., Kearney, J.F., Lawton, A.R., and M.D. Cooper. 1978. Pre-B cells. Bone marrow persistance in anti-u suppressed mice, conversion to B lymphocytes and recovery after destruction by cyclophosmamide.

11. Fenner, M., Frischknecht, H., Binz. H., Lindenmann, H., and H. Wigzell. 1979. Alloantigens derived from stimulator cells and bound to MLC-activated rat T lymphoblasts. Scand.J.Immunol. 9: 553.

12. Binz. H., Frischknecht, H., Mercilli, C., Dunst, S., and H. Wigzell. 1979. Binding of purified, soluble MHC polypeptide chains onto isolated T cell receptors. I. Reactivity against allo-and self-determinants. J.Exp.Med. 150: 1084.

13. Strong, D.M., Ahmed, A., Leapman, S.B., Gawith, K., Goldman, M.H., Smit, A.H. and K.W. Sell. 1979. Induction of memory cells in vitro with an antiidiotype serum against recognition structure specific for cells primed for histocompatibility determinants. Transplant.Proc. 11:928.

Synthesizing an immunologic circuit

Harvey Cantor and Richard K.Gershon*

Harvard Medical School/Farber Cancer Institute and *Howard Hughes Medical Institute Laboratory, Yale University Medical School

ABSTRACT

We describe here a general method for producing continuously propaga-table clones of immunologic cells that mediate one or another function. The procedure does not require hybridization to tumor cells. It is based upon the finding that (a) each set of T or non-T cells requires different physio-logic signals to potentiate in vitro growth and maintain antigen-specific regulatory function and (b) long term stimulation of unselected, heterogen-eous cell suspensions results in suppressive interactions that inactivate antigen-specific function after a short period of time (with the possible exception of T cells reactive to MHC products).

INTRODUCTION

T-cell Sets and Antibody Production

Stimulation of the immune system by almost any foreign material ("antigen") results in secretion of immunoglobulins that bind specifically to determinants carried on the antigen with an average affinity of greater than 10^5 M. Restimulation by the same antigen elicits higher serum levels of antibodies characterized by considerably higher binding affinities.[1,2]

We do not understand the series of cellular or molecular events that ensure production of specific antibodies after initial and secondary stimu-lation by antigen. The first notion that made sense was the "clonal selec-tion theory"[3] which simply assumed that the Darwinian rules that governed prokaryotic cells, as shown by the classical experiments of Luria and Del-bruck, might also apply to eukaryotic cells. According to this notion, each immunologic cell was genetically programmed to express, at its mem-brane surface, a single "receptor" molecule capable of binding to deter-minants composed of peptides or sugar residues. When an immunological cell made contact with a determinant that fit well with its receptor molecule, the cell multiplied rapidly, giving rise to a "clone" of thousands of daughter cells, each marked by the same surface receptor, each programmed to secrete a modified form of its surface receptor, antibody, into the

blood stream. Like populations of bacteria, the fittest immunologic cells
were <u>selected</u> to multiply: the configuration of immunoglobulins within
lymphocytes were not "imprinted" by small bits of ingested antigen.[4]

Despite the diversity of antibodies produced after stimulation of
immunologic cells, they do not normally secrete antibodies that bind to
molecules expressed on an individual's own tissues. According to the clonal
selection idea, this discrimination reflected elimination, during ontogeny,
of immunologic cells that bound to molecules expressed on an individual's
own tissues. Occasional severe "auto-immune" reactions were blamed upon
renegade cells that had somehow escaped elimination during development of
the immune system; these cells carried "forbidden" receptors that recognized "self" determinants. The subsequent finding that lymphocytes that
developed in the thymus ("T cells") were required to activate or "help"
antibody-forming cells ("B" lymphocytes) secrete antibodies[5,6] did not
alter this view; it meant that elimination of self-reactive clones from
either the T or B compartment would suffice to avoid autoimmune reactions.

Recent analyses of immunologic cells has supported a different view of
the immune system; discrimination between "self" and "non-self" reflects interactions among immunologic cell sets that are processed in the
thymus; the intensity, avidity and duration of immune responses are
determined by interactions among three major sets of immunologic cells--
inducer cells, regulatory cells, and effector cells. Although these cell
sets are morphologically indistinguishable, each is marked by surface
glycoproteins that are invariably expressed as part of the genetic program
that also determines the function of the set. Antibodies to these "marker"
glycoproteins have been used to identify, separate and analyze the role of
each set in the generation of antibody reactions <u>in vitro</u> and <u>in vivo</u>.[7]
The basic experimental strategy that has generated this view of the immune
system, as well as a summary of recent work that has begun to define the
genetic and molecular basis of communication among inducer, regulatory, and
effector immunologic cells has been recently reviewed.[8]

An experimental fact obtained from this approach is as follows:
The majority (about 60%) of T cells expressing a characteristic set of
surface glycoproteins (Ly1, Ly2, Ly3) in all mouse strains are not genetically equipped to induce ("help") B cells to secrete antibody, even after
hyperimmunization (Table I).

So, even after stimulation by antigen, the majority of cells in the
peripheral T cell pool (the Ly123 set) are unable to induce or "help" B

TABLE I
The Majority of T Cells are not Genetically Programmed to Help
B Cells Secrete Antibody

T Cell Set in SRBC-stimulated culture*	% of Total T cells in murine lymphoid tissues	B cells (10^6)	anti-SRBC PFC/culture
[Ly1]	30	+	1560
[Ly1$_i$]	30	+	6450
[Ly123]	65	+	112
[Ly123$_i$]	65	+	125
[Ly23$_i$]	5-10	+	96
None	−	+	105

*The indicated T cell sets were obtained after positive selection using monoclonal antibodies specific for Ly1, Ly2 or Ly3 cell surface determinants on T cells. After incubation x5 days with SRBC, anti-SRBC PFC were enumerated in triplicate cultures.

The subscript "i" indicates that the cells were obtained from donors immunized with 10^8 SRBC 1 week previously.

cells secrete antibody. What, then, is their function? A signal from Ly1 inducer T cells specifically activates a portion of Ly123 set to inhibit antigen specific T:B cooperation (Table II). These, and other data,[9-11] have demonstrated that, after activation by antigen, Ly1 inducer cells (a) activate B cells to secrete antibody and (b) stimulate a second set of T cells to directly inhibit Ly1 inducer activity. The outcome of this T-T interaction is a reduction in formation of antibody (by B cells) and decreased generation of suppression (by T cells). Further studies have shown

TABLE II
Suppression of Antibody Production by the Ly123 Set

T Cell Set in SRBC-stimulated culture*	B cells (10^6)	anti-SRBC PFC/culture
Ly1$_i$	+	6450
Ly1$_i$ + Ly123	+	550
Ly1$_i$ + Ly123$_i$	+	410
Ly1$_i$ + Ly23$_i$	+	690

*The indicated T cell sets were obtained after positive selection using monoclonal antibodies specific for Ly1, Ly2 or Ly3 cell surface determinants on T cells. After incubation x5 days with SRBC, anti-SRBC PFC were enumerated in triplicate cultures.

The subscript "i" indicates that the cells were obtained from donors immunized with 10^8 SRBC 1 week previously.

that this inducer:acceptor T-T interaction is highly specific and is mediated by gene products linked to the Ig-V_H locus.[12]

T Cell Clones

This inducer:acceptor T-T interaction generates highly specific T suppressor cells: addition of SRBC-stimulated Ly23[+] suppressor cells to cell cultures stimulated by both SRBC and HRBC results in inhibition of the PFC response to the former but not the latter erythrocyte.[13] However, the molecules responsible for antigen-specific recognition and the associated "constant region" that determines suppression or help have not been defined. Biochemical definition of the subunits of the immunoglobulin molecule responsible for antibody function and specificity has depended on the availability of amounts of homogeneous immunoglobulin molecules secreted by neoplastic clones of B cells--myeloma cells.[14-16] Similar analysis of the molecular basis of the specificity and function of different T cell sets has not been possible because methods for obtaining large amounts of homogeneous, antigen-specific functional T cells are not available.

"T cell" lymphomas have not proved as useful as myelomas. Continuous activation of T cells by supernatants of Con A-stimulated spleen cells have not resulted in efficient growth of antigen-specific T cell clones that secrete relevant molecules in significant amounts. "Hybrids" formed after fusion of T cells to T cell tumors rarely develop and maintain specific T cell function (perhaps due to continuous chromosome loss). Moreover, greater than 95% of the proteins secreted by "positive" hybridomas represent products of the tumor cell partner (G. Nabel and H. Cantor, in preparation).

We describe here a general method for producing continuously propagatable clones of immunologic cells that mediate one or another function. The procedure does not require hybridization to tumor cells. It is based upon the finding that (a) each set of T or non-T cells requires different physiologic signals to potentiate in vitro growth and maintain antigen-specific regulatory function and (b) long term stimulation of unselected, heterogeneous cell suspensions results in suppressive interactions that inactivate antigen-specific function after a short period of time (with the possible exception of T cells reactive to MHC products).

This method allows (a) preselection of the particular T cell set to be studied (e.g., TL[+] thymocytes, suppressor precursor, suppressor effector, and inducer T cell sets), (b) preselection of the specificity of the T cell set that is to be clonally expanded and (c) generation of large numbers of

continuously propagatable clones of non-transformed cells that are specialized to synthesize and secrete functionally active, antigen-specific
polypeptides which represent between 5-10% of the total proteins synthesized
by these T cell clones, and greater than 80% of the total secreted polypeptides.

So far, we have defined conditions that allow clonal growth of prothymocytes, thymocytes, antigen-specific T inducer (helper) cells, "natural
killer" cells and antigen-specific, mature T suppressor cells (G. Nabel,
A. Chessman, M. Fresno and H. Cantor, ms. in preparation). We describe
here the approach taken to generate clones of $Ly23^+$ "mature" T suppressor
cells to secrete substantial amounts of antigen-specific polypeptides.

RESULTS

Antigen

T cell clones secreting receptors that bind to either TNP or glycophorin
from sheep erythrocytes have been produced. This article will outline the
procedure for generation of glycophorin specific Ts clones. The advantages
of SRBC as antigen are as follows: (a) the in vitro bioassay for SRBC-
specific T suppression is simple, reproducible and has been used extensively
in our laboratories to characterize regulatory interactions among T cell
sets;[8] (b) since the presence of antigen is required to stimulate clonal
growth of Ts cells in culture, the sheep erythrocyte is attractive because
high concentrations of this material, unlike many other antigens, are non-
toxic in long-term in vitro cultures; (c) after immunization in vivo with
sheep erythrocytes, as judged by rosette formation, all antigen binding T
cells are $Ly2^+$ (Table III);[17] (d) although SRBC is not a homogeneous antigen,
70-80% of T cells that bind to SRBC are inhibited by glycophorin (a major
erythrocyte glycoprotein) from sheep, but not horse, human or rat erythrocytes; (e) M. Iverson has defined a cross-reactive idiotype (CRI_s) present
on 60-80% of early IgM anti-SRBC antibodies that is also expressed on SRBC-
specific $Ly2^+$ T cells (Table III); (f) since almost all of these "T-RFC" are
$Ly2^+$, SRBC specific T suppressor cells can be substantially enriched after
elution from plates coated with sheep, but not horse or human glycophorin
(Table IV).

TABLE III

Inhibition of T Cells that Bind Sheep Erythrocytes

Material included during T-RFC formation	No. SRBC-specific T-RFC/10^6 Cells[a]	
	SRBC-immune T cells	CRBC-immune[b] T cells
None	6500	50
Sheep erythrocyte glycophorin (1 mcg/ml)	950	ND
Human erythrocyte glycophorin (1 mcg/ml)	7300	ND
anti-CRI$_s$[c]	600	ND
anti-DRI$_s$[d]	6800	ND

[a] T-RFC = Thy1$^+$ cells (obtained from donors immunized with 10^8 sheep erythrocytes [SRBC] 1 wk previously) that bind >5 SRBC/cell; 88% of T-RFC are Ly2$^+$.

[b] Thy1$^+$ cells obtained from donors immunized with 10^8 chicken erythrocytes (CRBC).

[c] Ig fraction of anti-CRI$_s$ after passage through sepharose columns coated with anti-HRBC antibodies; final concentration during T-RFC formation = 1:200.

[d] Ig fraction of anti-CRI$_s$ after passage through sepharose columns coated with anti-SRBC antibodies; final concentration during T-RFC formation = 1:200.

TABLE IV
Enrichment of Glycophorin-Binding Ts Cells

Glycophorin coated plate	No. of adherent Ly2$^+$ cells/10^6 applied*	% suppression of α-SRBC PFC response by 10^4 eluted cells
Sheep erythrocyte	2-8x10^4	90
Human erythrocyte	2-6x10^2	0 (+10)
Horse erythrocyte	4-9x10^2	5

*Donors = mice immunized with 10^8 SRBC 1 wk earlier.

Definition of Cell Supernatant Material Required for Optimal Induction and Continued Expression of Ly23$^+$ Antigen-specific Suppressive Activity

(1) Lyl:Qal$^+$ inducer cells are required for generation and expression of Ly23$^+$ antigen-specific Ts activity. Ly23 cells from SRBC-primed donors are restimulated in vitro with SRBC and tested for their ability to suppress primary in vitro anti-erythrocyte responses. Stimulation of isolated Ly23 cells in the presence of Lyl:Qal$^+$ inducer cells from primed donors generated

maximal amounts of Ly23 SRBC-specific suppression[18] (also Eardley, Shen, Cantor and Gershon, ms. submitted for publication).

(2) Supernatants of SRBC-stimulated Ly1 cells from donors identical at the Ig locus are required for optimal induction and expression of Ly23-mediated suppressive activity. Because generation of maximal antigen-specific suppressive activity from Ly23 cells requires induction by Ly1 inducer cells, we asked whether supernates of SRBC-stimulated Ly1 cells might mimic the activity of intact Ly1 inducer cells, and therefore could be used to potentiate specific clonal growth of antigen-specific Ly23 Ts cells (Table V).

(3) Definition of the genetic requirements for production of maximal inducer activity. The ability of Ly1 supernates to activate Ly23 Ts cells was abolished if small amounts of anti-CRI_s was included in Ly23 cultures (data not shown). This observation, and others,[12] suggested the possibility that inducer supernatants were efficient only if obtained from Ly1 cells that expressed Ig V_H genes identical to $Ly2^+$ Ts acceptor cells. This proved to be the case: supernates from SRBC-primed inducer cells from donors that differed from Ly23 acceptor cells at the Ig V_H locus were unable to directly activate Ly23-mediated SRBC-specific suppressive activity (Yamauchi, Shen, Cantor and Gershon, Ms. in preparation).

(4) Requirements for continued expression of Ly23 Ts activity in long-term culture. Analysis of the in vitro conditions necessary to expand clones of Ly23 cells that expressed SRBC-specific suppression indicated the following: (a) continuous presence of antigen in culture, (b) a "feeder

TABLE V
Ly1 Inducer Supernatants Activate Antigen-Specific $Ly2^+$ T Suppression

*Supernates of Ly1 cells from donors immunized to:		% Suppression**			
SRBC	HRBC	PFC response/ culture after stimulation of T + B cells with SRBC	PFC response/ culture after stimulation of T + B cells with HRBC	PFC response/ culture after stimulation of Ly1 + B cells with SRBC	PFC response/ culture after stimulation of Ly1 + B cells with HRBC
	+	0	78	0	0
+		86	5	3	3

*B6 mice were immunized at day 0 and day 14 with either 10' SRBC or HRBC i.v.; after sacrifice at day 28, Ly1 cells were obtained from spleen and incubated x48 hrs in RPMI 1640 media + 2% FCS. Supernatants were obtained after 10,000 g centrifugation and added to RBC stimulated assay cultures at a final dilution of 1:100.

**Control anti-SRBC PFC response/culture = 1190±87
Control anti-HRBC PFC response/culture = 880±40

layer" consisting of irradiated spleen cells pretreated with anti-Ly2 and complement, (c) addition, every other day, of "inducer" supernatants (obtained from cultures containing spleen cells depleted of $Ly2^+$ cells from donors immunized to SRBC supplemented with 15% FCS. Small amounts of Con A (.5 mcg/ml) present in inducer supernates are removed after passage through sephadex G-50 columns and (d) culture media consisting of Dulbecco's modified Eagles media supplemented with a 10-fold excess of non-essential amino acids.

Production of $Ly23^+$ Ts Clones*

(1) Cloning. T cells from B6 mice immunized with SRBC 5 days earlier are incubated on plates coated with sheep erythrocyte glycophorin. Adherent cells are distributed into microwells at a final concentration of 1-10 cells per well. Initially, each well contains (a) a feeder layer of irradiated anti-Ly2 + C treated spleen cells and (b) Dulbecco's modified Eagles media containing a 10-fold excess of non-essential amino acids supplemented with inducer supernatant. This procedure results in a cloning efficiency that ranges between from 30-70%. After initial growth, cloned cells can be grown in vitro in the absence of feeder layer spleen cells.

(2) Screening for positive clones. Ten to 14 days after initiation of growth, cultures are pulsed with ^{35}S methionine x2 hrs; supernatants are tested for ability to bind to (a) sheep, horse, or human glycophorin and (b) ability to inhibit mixtures of Lyl cells and B cells to secrete anti-SRBC antibody in vitro. Testing of supernatants in assay cell cultures containing purified Lyl inducer ("helper") cells and B cells is critical: supernatants that specifically suppress this response contain polypeptides that directly inhibit T_H:B cell collaboration, and secrete substantially larger amounts of antigen-specific material than clones of $Ly23^+$ cells that do not directly suppress the T_H:B interaction, but activate $Ly2^+$ cells in assay cultures to develop inhibitor activity. A clone is considered "positive" if ^{35}S-labelled supernatant binds to sheep but not horse or human glycophorin, and SRBC-specific inhibitory activity is removed after incubation of the supernatant on petri dishes coated with sheep but not horse or human erythrocyte glycophorin.

A more efficient screening assay that has the advantage of defining large numbers of clones that actively secrete antigen-specific suppressive molecules depends on the use of a serum from rabbits immunized to suppressor factor that inhibits contact sensitivity responses. This material is ob-

---

*G. Nabel, A. Chessman, and H. Cantor, ms. in preparation.

tained from supernatants of _in vitro_ cultures of Lyl and Ly23 cells as a
result of a T-T interaction: Lyl inducer cells obtained from picryl chloride
painted donors simulate Ly2$^+$ cells from TNBS-injected donors to produce
suppressive material (MW $\sim$70,000) during a 2-day culture period. These
polypeptides inhibit T cell mediated transfer of contact sensitivity to
TNCB. Suppressive activity is depleted after passage through TNP (but not
DNP or oxazalone)-coated sepharose columns and is enriched in the column-
elute (after elution with excess TNP-lysine). After dialysis, this TNP
"affinity purified" material is administered in CFA to rabbits. The resultant sera does not react with mouse immunoglobulins, anti-TNP antibodies,
fetal calf sera or DNP; it binds to determinants expressed on the "constant"
region of molecules secreted by T cells that suppress both cellular and
T-dependent antibody reactions to a variety of antigens (Ptak, Cone, Rosen-
stein, Boudreau, Cantor and Gershon, Ms. in preparation).

For example, addition of DEAE purified Ig fraction of rabbit "anti-
TSF" to cell cultures stimulated with sheep or horse erythrocytes, results
in 10-50 fold increase in anti-RBC PFC production; addition to cultures of
T cells stimulated with chemically modified syngeneic cells or allogeneic
cells results in a 5-25 fold enhancement of the CTL response. In both
cases, preincubation of "anti-TSF" with Ig$^-$ but not Ig$^+$ cells removes
enhancing activity.

Although analysis of the mechanism of anti-TSF potentiation of immunity
is the major object of current experiments, it has also proved useful as
a "developing" reagent to identify clones of T cells that secrete SRBC-
specific suppressive molecules (using the Cunningham modification of the
Jerne plaque assay) and should provide a rapid and sensitive screen for
T cell clones that secrete suppressive molecules specific for antigens that
can be conjugated to erythrocytes.

(3) Verification of clonal growth. The clonal nature of cell growth
is verified in each experiment by analyzing the progeny of 50:50 mixtures of
cells from male and female B6 donors. After 14 days, 100 wells or more
are stimulated with Con A and the presence or absence of the Y chromosome is
determined from metaphase preparations after stimulation. Testing of cultures seeded initially with approximately 1-10 cells/well has indicated
that, in the large majority of experiments, no wells contain a mixture of
male and female cells. In addition, cell cultures producing positive
supernates are recloned using the above criteria to ensure that the cellular
source of positive supernatants is a clonal.

More recently, recloning of cells from "positive" wells is accomplished by transfer of single cells, using micromanipulation techniques. Despite their rapid in vitro growth (doubling time: 14-24 hrs), it is unlikely that these clones are "tumors". Neither recloning nor continuous long-term growth (up to 5 months) has, so far, resulted in loss of specific immunologic function. They require the continuous presence of antigen and Lyl inducer supernatant for continued in vitro growth; they do not form tumors after injection into syngeneic irradiated or unirradiated hosts; and karyotypic analysis of the chromosomes of several clones has not revealed any quantitative or qualitative abnormalities.

Characterization of an Antigen-specific T Suppressor Clone

(1) T-21 (surface phenotype: $Thyl^+Lyl^-Ly23^+Ig^-$).* T-21 cultures are pulsed x2 hrs with ^{35}S-Methionine, centrifuged x1/2 hr at 10,000 G and incubated at 4 C on plates coated with glycophorin from sheep, horse or human RBC. No significant binding to horse or human glycophorin is detected, as judged by amount of radioactivity bound to the plate after extensive washing. By contrast, plates coated with sheep glycophorin contained substantial amounts of ^{35}S-labelled material, representing greater than 80% of the secreted material. SDS polyacrylamide gel analysis of the internally labelled material (after elution from antigen-coated plates) indicates a single polypeptide having an apparent molecular weight of 68,000 d. It is likely that the T-21 68,000 d polypeptide that binds to SRBC glycophorin represents a single moiety with specificity for SRBC glycophorin in view of the clonal source of the material and the restricted acrylamide gel pattern (Figure 1).

DISCUSSION

Cellular immunology has, for the most part, represented a catalogue of phenomena mediated by lymphocytes that are not understood in molecular terms. More recently, the diverse regulatory and effector functions mediated by morphologically indistinguishable lymphocytes have been assigned to T cell sets that each express different genetic programs combining information for immune function (e.g., inducer activity, suppressor activity) and expression of a unique set of marker glycoproteins on their cell membrane.[7] A similar approach has been taken in man and has defined analogous regulatory T cell sets.[19] Nonetheless, the molecular basis of these specific

*A detailed description of methodology for generation of cloned lymphocyte sets and characterization of their antigen-binding polypeptides is in preparation--G. Nabel, M. Fresno, A. Chessman, and H. Cantor.

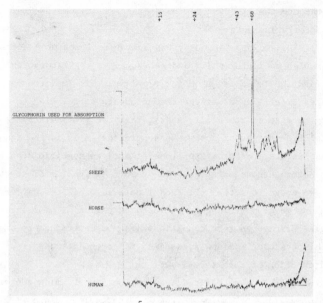

Figure 1. Cultures containing 2×10^5 T-21 cells in Methionine-free Eagle's media, supplemented with dialyzed 1% fetal calf serum, were incubated x2 hrs with 200 microcuries of ^{35}S-methionine. The supernatants were collected and centrifuged (10,000 g x1/2 hr). Aliquots of the spun supernatant, containing approximately 20,500 cpm each, were applied to dishes coated with sheep, horse and human erythrocyte glycophorin. After extensive washing, approximately 16,000 cpm were bound to plates coated with sheep glycophorin, compared with 1950 and 900 cpm after incubation of the super-natants on dishes coated with horse or human glycophorin. The labelled material was eluted under high salt conditions (4M KCl in PBS) and loaded onto a 15% acrylamide slab gel under reducing conditions at 60 volts/hr. After DMSO treatment (20% PPO) x3 hrs, the gel was dried and exposed x3 days. Densitometry scans of the three gels are shown.

T cell functions is unknown. By contrast, the biochemical basis of the function and specificity of antibodies has been precisely defined using myelomas in mouse[14] and in man[15] as a source of large amounts of homogeneous immunoglobulins.

An analogous effort has been made to define the molecules responsible for antigen specific T cell functions. Unfortunately, "T cell lymphomas" have not proved as useful as neoplastic B cells: they do not secrete antigen specific functional molecules. In addition, efforts to immortalize normal T cells by fusion with T cell tumors have been, on the whole, dis-appointing. Except for one or two cases, the hybrid expresses the phenotype of the tumor partner, rapidly loses chromosomes, and there is no published biochemical data defining the molecule(s) secreted by a cloned "hybrid". It is possible that identification of a more stable, differentiated T cell tumor than the one that is commonly used (the AKR thymoma BW-5147) may yield more encouraging data.

Our efforts to grow continuously propagatable clones of T cells that secrete molecules mediating their antigen-specific regulatory function have identified the following as major problems: (1) In vitro expansion of unseparated T cells from antigen-primed donors before cloning is unsatisfactory because inducer cells specifically activate T suppressor cells. Since one cellular target of activated suppressor cells is the inducer cell itself, this results in concomitant loss of antigen-specific suppressor cell activity in heterogeneous cultures. The result is functional inactivation of all antigen specific sets. (2) Each T cell set requires different culture conditions to support long-term cloned expansion without loss of function. The precise culture conditions must be determined by analysis of the normal physiologic signals required to potentiate the growth and specialized function of each T cell set.

In this article we have defined the protocols that allow continuous propagation of a clone belonging to the Ly23 set. This clone (T-21) secretes a polypeptide that specifically suppresses the interaction between T inducer cells and B cells. Although the requirements for clonal expansion of mature (Ly23$^+$) T suppressor cells have been studied in most detail, in vitro culture conditions allowing clonal expansion of at least certain types of Ly1 T inducer cells, TL$^+$ thymocytes and "natural killer" cells have been developed. Analysis of cloned immunologic cells (and their products) that carry specific immunologic function represents a central approach to understanding cellular regulation of the immune system, and cellular differentiation in higher organs.

"Immunoregulation"

An enormous amount of experimental analyses have been undertaken in the past few years to clarify the sequence of events that regulate production of specific antibodies. The general strategy is to determine the effect of various manipulations of heterogeneous populations of immunologic cells upon the quantity and quality of immune responses.

Individual T cell clones expressing a defined antigen-specific immunoregulatory activity represent highly attractive material for biochemical analysis. But there is an additional major point that can be made from close examination of cell-cell interactions between clones of T cells expressing defined function and specificity. Production of clones of antigen-specific functional T cells might allow a synthetic, rather than a reduc-

tionist, approach to understanding the cellular and molecular basis of
cell-cell interactions that govern the immune response. This strategy
depends on "building" or synthesizing the minimal cloned sets required for
a specific immune response, supplemented by populations of B cells and
different sets of antigen-presenting cells. The predictive value of propo-
sitions that have derived from reductionist analysis of the immune system
can then be stringently tested.

(1) Application of defined, clonally expanded T cell sets to understanding cell-cell interactions. T"help": Secretion of antibody requires
an "interaction" among thymus-processed lymphocytes and lymphocytes that
differentiate elsewhere. The mechanism of this interaction is not clear.
How do antigen-stimulated T inducer cells locate and trigger the "correct"
clone of (antigen-specific) B cells? Do T inducer cells bear a receptor
for an antigen (perhaps associated in some way with H-2 linked gene products?
Does efficient B cell activation require a second inducer cell specific for
idiotypic determinants on the B cell receptor?[20] This can be approached by
analysis of clones to Ly1 inducer cells required to activate id$^+$ B cells
to secrete id$^+$ antibody. Finally, can one identify and quantitate clones of
Ly23 cells that specifically inhibit this inducer:B cell induction, and
isolate the cellular target of clonal suppression?

"MHC" structures and the T cell receptor for antigen: There is increasing evidence that T inducer cells (Ly1 cells) recognize antigen in
association with MHC (probably I region) coded determinants. These findings
have given rise to the notion that Ly1 "T_H" cells recognize conventional
antigen ("X") in association with self MHC products using a single receptor
which recognizes a neo-antigenic determinant formed by juxtaposition of an
MHC product + X, or two receptors having specificity for the host's MHC
products and X, respectively. There is no definitive evidence to support
either model.

According to a "one receptor" model for T cell recognition, it must be
presumed that the restricting MHC structure makes a significant contribution
to the affinity of binding of the T cell receptors for antigen. Using, for
example, an Ly1 "T-33" type clone, one can ask whether those cells can be
activated by glycophorin-pulsed macrophages that are matched or mismatched
at the MHC locus. The proliferative response of a single Ly1 clone should
not be confounded by "allogeneic" effects which can be, in any event,
ruled out using unpulsed allogeneic macrophages. If no MHC restriction is
observed, this would provide strong evidence that a portion of Ly1 inducer

cells carry receptors for antigenic determinants, as do B cells, and lack affinity for MHC-specified structures. If MHC restriction is apparent, this would favor contribution of MHC products to binding by a T cell clone. Either model could then be directly tested by analysis of the biochemical and binding properties of T cell receptor material obtained after stimulation of cloned Ly1 cells by antigen-pulsed macrophages.

An extraordinarily large number of T cells respond to alloantigens (as judged by mixed lymphocyte reactions of mouse, rat and human cells). The frequency of reactive cells after stimulation across a single MHC haplotype difference has been estimated at approximately 4-8%. Similarly, the frequency of prekiller cells in the Ly23 population capable of developing into cytotoxic effector cells act as such stimulation has been estimated at approximately 2-4%. Since haplotypes of "independent" origin probably do not cross-react to a mean level greater than about 20%, it is difficult to accomodate all allogeneic reactions in mice in less than about 70% of the T cell pool.

Taken together, these observations imply the presence of an extraordinarily large number of alloreactive cells in the T cell population. This apparent commitment of T cells to specificities expressed by polymorphic variants of the MHC ("alloaggression") has puzzled immunologists because of the apparent biologic irrelevance of immunity to foreign MHC products. In addition, it has raised the issue of whether clones of T cells that react to alloantigens represent a separate and distinguishable set from those that recognize conventional antigens or whether reactivity is mediated by the same clones (which normally, for example, react to conventional antigens associated with self-MHC products, and "cross-react" with polymorphic variants of the MHC).

At present there is no direct method for demonstrating the separate existence of a pool of cells programmed to respond to conventional antigen (in association with self-MHC) and a pool recognizing polymorphic variants of the MHC. A direct approach to this question can be formulated as follows: a T_H clone (e.g., T-33) specific for a conventional antigen (e.g., SRBC) can be tested for proliferative reactivity against a panel of cells expressing different MHC haplotypes. Reactivation can be measured either by increase in ^{3}H-T incorporation in cultures supplemented with 2% rat sera to induce "background" ^{3}H-T levels, or for ability to help Ly23 cells generate cytotoxic effector activity. If such reactivity is found, it will be highly selective; that is, directed against no more than one foreign MHC haplotype.

If this is the case, one can determine whether the ability of the clone to react to foreign MHC antigens reflects recognition by <u>different</u> or identical binding sites.

(2) Polypeptides secreted by T cell clones. <u>H-2 restricted cytotoxic cells</u>: Maximal cytotoxic reactions (in vitro) occur only if virus-infected target cells display H-2K or H-2D gene products identical to the H-2K or D products expressed by virus-infected cells that first stimulated T killer cells. This phenomenon, called "H-2 restriction", is thought to imply that the specificities of T killer cells include recognition of "self marking" H-2 molecules: this functional specificity might reflect surface receptor molecules consisting of <u>one</u> binding site specific for a "neoantigen" formed by intimate association between a viral antigen and a H-2K or H-2D molecule. Alternatively, this phenomenon might indicate that killer cells bear two distinct binding sites: one specific for the host's H-2K or H-2D products and a second for the foreign antigen. Occupation of both is necessary to trigger the cytotoxic cell to kill. There is no data that rules out either molecular explanation. We have developed clones of CTL specific for virus infected targets (e.g., expressing β-propriolactone-inactivated sendai virus and a Moloney transformed lymphoma). Sufficient amounts of internally labelled peptide can be obtained that specifically bind target cells (interestingly, the majority of the material is purified from the membrane fraction of the clones and not secreted). Does binding reflect separate interactions of two distinct polypeptides? If not, is the affinity of binding to purified virus by a single polypeptide influenced by the appropriate purified H-2 molecules? Finally, will these polypeptides bind well to different MHC allelic products, providing a direct test of the molecular basis of "alloaggression"?

<u>MHC products on thymic stroma may determine T cell recognition</u>: The H-2 genotype of stem cells ("Pro-thymocyte") is irrelevant. For example, stem cells from, say, strain H-2^x that differentiate within an H-2^y thymus generate mature T cells that treat H-2^y (rather than H-2^x) as "self". These conclusions have come from experiments in which "lethally" irradiated inbred mice are (a) infused with bone marrow or fetal liver cells from donors differing at the MHC locus, or (b) thymectomized and implanted with an MHC-different (irradiated) thymus before infusion of bone marrow cells.

There are many variations on these two experimental themes. It is not yet possible to draw conclusions from these protocols, primarily because the experimental data from different laboratories differ for unexplained reasons. Production and analysis of the binding properties of peptides obtained from cloned prothymocyte and thymocyte lines that have been educated on feeder layer cells expressing defined MHC phenotypes represents a direct approach to this question.

Cellular Differentiation

Cellular differentiation in a complex organism like a mouse also connotes a series of absolute commitments that, step by step, dictate the production of the mature organism from the zygote formed at conception. In the following, it is implicit that genesis of several sets of diversely-programmed lymphocytes, probably from a single stem cell type, represents in miniature this entire process and, hence that mechanisms established by the study of this population of cells may prove applicable to cellular differentiation in general.

One can focus on a single differentiation step as a cell passes from one compartment into a succeeding compartment, and attempt to answer some of the following questions: Does this step reflect the result of an already prescribed program that brings into action a new set of genes, which in turn allows the expression of new functional properties? What is the nature of the inducing agent which is the physiologic signal for this program to be put into effect? Where does this signal come from? How is it delivered to the cell and how is its message transmitted from the cell surface to the nucleus? And, finally, can a single cell give rise to only one or more than one type of progeny? If the latter, does this "choice" depend upon the nature of the inducing signal?

What is the immediate common precursor of Ly1 inducer cells and Ly23 suppressor cells? The cell that has not yet realized one of its two (or more) mutually-exclusive options. A likely candidate is the TL^-Ly123 subclass or some member of it. Alternatively, all TL^-Ly123 cells might belong to a separate T cell lineage and all three TL^- T cell subclasses may be descended from TL^+Ly123^+ thymocytes. We currently favor the first model because we have found that after stimulation with chemically-altered syngeneic cells, some Ly123 cells give rise to Ly23 progeny[20] and Ly1 progeny (unpublished data).

We do not know whether these Ly1 and Ly23 cells are progeny of separate subpopulations of Ly123 cells, programmed to generate either Ly1 or Ly23 functional daughter cells after stimulation, or whether a single Ly123 cell can give rise to both cell sets. The answer to this question bears directly upon our understanding of cellular differentiation in higher organisms. Can a single cell give rise to only one or more than one type of progeny?   If the latter, does this "choice" depend upon the nature of the inducing signal?   We have succeeded in raising clones of Ly123$^+$ cells but have not defined their specificity for antigen.   These clones can be stimulated with a variety of inducing agents, including (a) supernatants of polyclonally-activated Ly1 and Ly23 cells, (b) agents thought to induce in vitro cellular differentiation such as insulin, protylytic enzymes, dibutryl cyclic AMP, cAMP agonists, FuDR or cGMP antagonists.[18]   For example, if these approaches indicate that a single clone of Ly123 cells can generate either progeny, the following additional question must be considered: Must the Ly123$^+$ clone proliferate to do so?   And if division is required, how does the Ly123 population maintain itself?   By unequal mitosis, i.e., Ly123→Ly123 + Ly1; alternative to Ly123→Ly123 + Ly23.   Or by equal mitosis, i.e., Ly123→Ly123 + Ly123; alternative to Ly123→Ly1 + Ly1; alternative to Ly123→Ly23 + Ly23. In addition, analysis of this differentiative step may allow definition of the inducing agent which is the physiologic signal for this new genetic program to be put into effect.   For example, do signals from Ly1 inducer cells activate Ly123→Ly23 differentiation?   What is the biochemical nature of the signal, is there a cell surface receptor for the inducer molecule? And, if so, how is the message transmitted from the cell surface to the nucleus after binding of the inducer molecule to the surface receptor?

Genetic mechanisms controlling B cell generation of antibody diversity: Recent experiments have used cloned DNA fragments from myeloma cells that control expression of the C and V regions of kappa and lambda light chains. Hybridization of these C-DNA probes to fragments of DNA obtained after restriction endonuclease treatment of DNA from other myelomas and DNA from "embryonic" tissues have led to the following hypothesis: (a) B cell differentiation is accompanied by a reduction in the length of the DNA sequence that intervenes between the structural V and C genes, and (b) light chain diversity is due to variation or mutation within DNA segments coding for "hypervariable" residues of the polypeptide.   These conclusions are not firmly established for two reasons: (1) Long-term lines of myeloma cells that have been passaged in vitro and in vivo for many years display marked karyotypic changes which may reflect deletional or translocational events resulting in abnormal or shortened DNA sequences that govern Ig secretion, compared to normal antibody-secreting B cells.   (2) Myeloma cells may represent a selected population of neoplastic B cells whose specificity has preserved for evolutionary reasons (e.g., because they carry genetic information coding for antibodies essential for immunologic protection of the organism). In this case, the genetic mechanisms operative in this set of B cells would serve to prevent normal physiological mechanisms of diversification.

As noted in the results section, glycophorin-specific T cell clones (a) do not exhibit karyotypic abnormalities and (b) require antigen for growth and secretion of substantial amounts of antigen-binding receptor material. These cells therefore represent more appropriate cellular material for analysis of the genetic events controlling the generation of immunologic diversity of thymus-processed lymphocytes.

Two approaches are currently being tested: (1) major RNA's of T-21 have been separated; preliminary analysis of one translated product suggests that the polypeptide binds to sheep glycophorin. The complementary DNA obtained from this major message can be produced by standard reverse transcription techniques. The DNA will be cloned and secreted products screened for T-21 protein. This cDNA probe can be incubated with restriction fragments obtained from (a) the T-21 clone, (b) T-33, a clone secreting a 68,000 dalton polypeptide that binds to TNP, and (c) cloned populations of thymocytes, prothymocytes and highly purified sperm. This approach should provide important information concerning the importance of rearrangement of DNA as a clone of cells differentiates from the "germ line" thymocytes, non-secreting lymphocytes, and secreting lymphocytes.

(2) An alternative approach is based on development of a panel of T cell clones that (a) bind to TNP, (b) secrete polypeptide that binds to TNP. One reacts with rabbit antibodies to the MOPC-315 idiotype. A cDNA probe made to the V_H region can be incubated with restriction fragments of DNA from (a) the clone secreting MOPC-315$^+$ DNP-binding material, (b) a second clone that is MOPC-315$^-$, (c) thymocyte clones, and (d) highly purified sperm. Analysis of the DNA sequence of the restriction fragments that bind to the MOPC-315 cDNA probe will indicate whether "gene arrangements" that are said to occur based upon a comparison of DNA from myeloma tumors to "embryonic tissue".

(3) Transformation of single cells: T-21 is not neoplastic (vide supra), despite the fact that it has been carried for 4 months in vitro. One might test whether the inclusion of purified materials that prevent expression of differentiated function of a single clone such as TPA might result in signs of transformation. The advantage of this approach is that one can monitor the effect of TPA by loss of differentiated function as well as chromosomal

change. The effect of TPA on non-cloned cell populations are difficult to interpret because some cells emit regulatory signals that induce normal differentiation in heterogeneous lymphoid populations and confound interpretation of the effects of "tumor promoters". That these regulatory cell-cell interactions that may normally prevent "transformation" may be illustrated by a so-called experiment of nature: the "MRL" mouse. Lyl inducer cells of this mouse strain lack a cell-surface receptor which normally receives regulatory signals from suppressor cells. These mice routinely develop an Lyl lymphoproliferative disorder, but, so far, these cells are not "fully" transformed: transfer into genetically identical inbred mice does not result in neoplasia. Clones of differentiated eukaryotic cells that can be tested for sequential loss of differentiated functions represent unique material for analysis of the biochemical events that lead, in stepwise fashion, to uncontrolled growth.

CONCLUSION

It is important to emphasize that no one can predict the impact of this method upon gaining a more penetrating view of the genetic and molecular basis of cellular differentiation. It is, however, certain that this technique will permit a more straightforward biochemical analysis of the differentiative events that lead to acquisition of immunological cells that differentiate in the thymus. Whether this technique will also provide an insight into the three major features of the immune system (absence of antibody reaction to individual's own tissues, generation and expression of antibody diversity, efficient and appropriate protection against bacterial and viral infection) remains to be tested.

There is also no doubt that the methodology described here will be improved and refined over the next several years. Nevertheless, it is certain that these technical improvements will depend upon the underlying principle of this method: Clonal expansion of immunologic cell sets specific for antigen will depend upon increased understanding of the normal physiologic signals required to potentiate the growth and specialized function of the individual T cell sets that comprise the immune system.

REFERENCES
1. Eisen, H.N. and G.W. Siskind. 1964. Variations in affinities of antibodies during the immune response. Biochemistry 3: 966
2. Kabat, E.A. 1976. Structural Concepts in Immunology and Immunochemistry. Holt, Rinehart and Winston Publishing Company, New York (2nd edition).
3. Burnet, F.M. 1959. The Clonal Selection Theory of Immunity. Vanderbilt University Press, Tennessee.
4. Haurowitz, F. 1968. Immunochemistry and the Biosynthesis of Antibodies. Interscience Publishers, New York

5. Claman, H.N., E.A. Chaperon and R.F. Triplett. 1966. Thymus-marrow cell combination-synergism in antibody production. Proc. Soc. Exp. Biol. Med. 122: 1167

6. Davies, A.J.S., J.H.L. Playfair, and A.M. Cross. Estimation in vivo of the viability of frozen and stored bone marrow. Transplantation 5:222

7. Cantor, H. and E.A. Boyse. 1977. Regulation of cellular and humoral immune response by T cell subclasses. In: Origin of Lymphocyte Diversity, Vol. 41, p 23, Cold Spring Harbor Laboratory, Cold Spring Harbor, New York.

8. Cantor, H. and R.K. Gershon. 1979. Immunological circuits: Cellular Composition. Federation Proceedings 38: 2058

9. Eardley, D.D., J. Hugenberger, L. McVay-Boudreau, F.W. Shen, R.K.Gershon and H. Cantor. 1978. Immunoregulatory circuits among T cell sets. I. T-helper cells induce other T-cell sets to exert feedback inhibition. J. Exp. Med. 147: 1106

10. Cantor, H., L. McVay-Boudreau, J. Hugenberger, K. Naidorf, F.W. Shen and R.K. Gershon. Immunoregulatory circuits among T cell sets. II. Physiologic role of feedback inhibition in vivo: Absence in NZB mice. J. Exp. Med. 147: 1116

11. Cantor, H., J. Hugenberger, L. McVay-Boudreau, D.D. Eardley, J. Kemp, F.W. Shen and R.K. Gershon. 1978. Immunoregulatory circuits among T cell sets: Identification of a subpopulation of T inducer cells that activates feedback inhibition. J. Exp. Med. 148: 871

12. Eardley, D.D., F.W.Shen, H.Cantor and R.K. Gershon. 1979. Genetic control of immunoregulatory circuits. Genes linked to the Ig locus govern communication between regulatory T-cell sets. J. Exp. Med. 150:44

13. Eardley, D.D. and R.K. Gershon. 1976. Induction of specific suppressor T cells in vitro. J..Immunol. 117: 313

14. Potter, M. 1972. Immunoglobulin-producing tumors and myeloma proteins of mice. Physiol. Rev. 52: 631

15. Natvig, J.B. and H. G. Kunkel. 1973. Human immunoglobulin: Classes, subclasses, genetics variance and idiotype. Adv. Immunol. 16:1

16. Edelman, G.M. 1971. Antibody structure in molecular immunology. Ann. NY Acad. Sci. 190:5

17. Eardley, D.D., F.W.Shen, R. Cone and R.K. Gershon. 1979. Antigen-binding T cells: Dose response and kinetic studies on the development of different subsets. J. Immunol. 122:140

18. Pollack, R. 1973. Readings of the Mammalian Cell in Culture. Cold Spring Harbor Press, Cold Spring Harbor, New York.

19. Reinherz, E.L. and S.F. Schlossman. 1979. Characteristics of regulatory T cells in man. In: Regulatory T Cells. (B.Pernis and H.Vogel, eds) Academic Press, New York

20. Woodland, R.T. and H. Cantor. 1978. Idiotype-specific T helper cells are required to induce idiotype-positive B memory cells to secrete antibody. Eur. J. Immunol. 8:600

SESSION III

Summary of Discussion

The session opened with a state-of-the-art review on the regulation of cellular events in allograft rejection. It was evident that the mechanisms by which cells cause rejection are still poorly understood, Mitchison's observations dating back some 25 years still are at the center of current thought. In this work rejection was shown to be produced by small numbers of leukocytes, whereas in the humoral immune system large volumes of antibody containing sera are required. While within rejected tissue dense infiltrations of mononuclear cells are seen, apparently only a fraction of these have specificity of action. The belief that contact between effector and target cells as a requirement for rejection has not been supplemented by fundamentally new observations. However, in vitro models demonstrate that requirements for allograft rejection may include immunologically specific T-effector cells, contact of the cells with target allogeneic cells, and sparing of "bystander" cells.

Attention was then called to some new experimental work suggesting that intimate contact between specific effector cells and target cells may not be an actual requirement for allogeneic rejection in in vivo situations (Winn). Transplantation of A/J skin to LAF_1 mice with retransplantation back to A/J mouse skin provided the basic model. After 15 days, the transplanted graft epidermis and vascular endothelium are still both of A/J origin. However, the 50 day grafts, though still of A/J epidermal composition, have vascular endothelium of LAF_1 origin and are subsequently rejected upon retransplantation to the A/J mouse. Because of these uncertainties pertaining to allograft rejection, it is believed that an avascular site such as the cornea could provide an opportune model for extended studies.

Discussion then centered on the possible role of blood supply and its inhibition in the process of graft rejection. The observation that immune rejection processes take place at a distance and cause cell death by blocking blood flow creates difficulty in the identification of those cells directly affected by the rejection mechanism. In turn, pertinent investigation in graft death is hampered. Here again, possible use of the avascular cornea as a useful tool to investigate the role of blood supply in organ rejection was pointed out.

The role of passenger leukocytes in graft rejection was next addressed. Since experimental work demonstrates that the antigenicity of passenger leukocytes is one determinant of the fate of a whole grafted organ, the presence of allogeneic leukocytes in syngeneic tissue may be responsible for rejection of an entire organ. Studies with thyroid grafts offer similar data with the additional unique finding that grafted thyroid parenchyma shows structural and functional recovery following rejection.

Other data support the concept that delayed type hypersensitivity (DTH) is a major factor in rejection reactions, whereas antibodies play only a minor role if at all. In regard to possible activity of cytotoxic lymphocytes in the rejection process, the belief was expressed that the inflammatory reaction triggered by DTH responses is more important than the more specific cytotoxic reaction. It was then pointed out that antibodies must play some important role in the inflammatory process accompanying DTH since the passive transfer of cells alone provokes reactions inferior to those effected by transfer of both cells and antibody. It is commonly believed that acute rejection episodes involve infiltration

by T cells whereas chronic rejection, which tends to be inexorable is
mediated by antibody, specifically antibody to the vascular endothelium of
the graft.

Discussion was initiated regarding the details and methods (reported
by Simmons for the University of Minnesota group) aimed at utilizing
all available kidneys. As a result of this emphasis, HLA matches for
only 0-2 antigens are obtained with very few for three and none for
four antigens. Additionally, in their experience results have been
the opposite of those reported by Kissmeyer-Nielsen in that recipients
of foreign HLA Ia antigens have actually demonstrated a higher degree of
graft survival.

Questions then arose concerning the current debate regarding the basis
of beneficial effects of prior blood transfusions in the aggregate. It is
not known whether transfusion exerts a real or only a selecting-out
effect. It is possible that genetically predisposed high responders would
react to transfusion by producing a high level of antibodies detectable in
subsequent matching. Thus, those sensitized by prior transfusion and
likely to be strong reactors will be ruled out for transplantation and in
turn alter the statistics. The real problem is that recipients might be
so responsive that one could never find a suitable kidney because of the
sensitizing effect of prior transfusion.

Regarding the use of a new drug agent, cyclosporin A, emerging data
(Calne) are sufficiently encouraging to warrant extended trial. While the
problem of side effects remains to be clarified, it does appear that
toxicity may cause little or no problem in recipients in which graft
kidneys function well immediately post-operatively.

Methods for the modification of graft antigeneticity by organ culture
especially in conjunction with high levels of oxygen were reviewed. The
objective is to effect macrophage and lymphocyte death at an accelerated

rate, leaving behind just non-inciting epithelial and fibroblastic allograft elements. Several organs including ovary, thyroid, pancreatic islets, parathyroids and thymus have been successfully transplanted by this approach. Adaptation of pre-transplantation organ culture to corneal tissue results in prolonged survival of xenografts from the chicken, guinea pig and human into rabbits, but allografts are not protected to the same degree. It was agreed that xenograft rejection is markedly different both quantitatively and qualitatively from allograft rejection and that data from one system cannot be extrapolated to the other; and it is expected that different immune mechanisms will be found to be involved in their respective rejections. In support of this concept, an experiment was noted in which autologous cornea immersed in ovalbumin prior to grafting results in cornea clouding due to an immune mechanism that is presumably different from the one responsible for rejection of the corneal allograft.

Modification of host responsiveness by passive treatment with antibody specific for the antigen to be grafted was reviewed and evidence offered that this procedure can alter both antibody production and CMI responses, including allograft enhancement by the host.

Efforts to obtain monoclonal antibodies to subsets of lymphocytes was reported (by the University of Chicago group) with data indicating cross reactions with lymphocytes from other subsets as well as from other species. Technical details have indicated an efficient fusion process with about 80 percent of cultured wells giving positive results with stability of hybridomas and minimal chromosomal loss. Wide cross reactivity could be explained on the basis of sugars common to immunizing cells and others of the lymphoid series.

It is anticipated that ongoing work with hybridomas will provide elegant techniques for both insight on mechanisms and for possible practical applications.

Regarding the possible use of hybridomas for production of antibodies to idiotypes, it was noted that definitive testing has not yet been accomplished. However, there is just a possible chance that this could be feasible with the technology currently available.

Inquiry was made into the subject of cross-reactivity between anti-idiotype molecules on T and B cells. It was noted that anti-idiotype sera produced by immunization with B cell products may react with T cell products. The frequency of this reaction is low but it can be increased by using for immunization B cell heavy chain. Additionally, antisera raised against T cell products may cross-react with B cell heavy chain. Though information on the existence of idiotype components specific for T or B cells is not definitive, it is believed that they may exist. The heterogeneity of anti-idiotype was emphasized in that idiotypes are present in high concentrations on lymphocytes which are demonstrable by gel precipitation reactions with antisera. Though isoelectric focusing has shown dominating bands, the exact number is not yet known.

Discussion was then directed to recent findings regarding "circuits" which comprise mechanisms for regulation of the immune system. The belief was expressed that the differing reports on helper cells carrying IJ markers (Tada; Feldman) may be due to the use of different investigative methods from those employed by Gershon (lack of effect of anti-IJ sera on helper cells in the sheep RBC system).

A simple and efficient method to obtain anti-idiotype sera was reported that is based upon immunization of sheep with sheep RBC coated with antibodies to this antigen that are raised in mice. Here, data demonstrated the blocking of 80-100 percent of the sheep RBC-binding T cells that bind these sheep RBC and that the location of idiotype B is on Ly 1 cells.

SESSION IV

IMMUNOLOGY OF TISSUE TRANSPLANTATION

Moderator: Arthur M. Silverstein

Ocular tumor immunology

Devron H.Char, M.D.

Ocular Oncology Unit, Department of Ophthalmology and Francis I. Procter Foundation,
University of California, San Francisco

ABSTRACT

The importance of immunologic phenomena in the human host-tumor interaction is unclear. In both retinoblastoma and choroidal melanoma immunologic
reactivity towards tumor-associated antigens has been demonstrated. The clinical efficacy of immunologic tests in ocular oncology is limited. These
tests may be useful diagnostically in the differentiation of primary choroidal
melanoma from choroidal metastases, and in the differentiation of orbital
lymphoid tumefaction. Possibly immune complex assays may be useful prognostically.

More work must be done to understand the importance of immunologic factors and immunologic mechanisms in ocular malignancies. Until this is accomplished, it will be impossible to develop a rational basis for immunotherapy.

INTRODUCTION

Immunologic alterations have been demonstrated in patients with both systemic and ocular malignancies; their biologic significance and potential vis-
a-vis human immunotherapy are uncertain. This brief review decribes the status
of immunologic research on eye tumors and its potential impact on immunotherapy in the management of these malignancies.

There are a number of clinical and pathologic observations which are consistent with the hypothesis that the immune system may be important in ocular
neoplasms. 1. Spontaneous remissions and regressions have been documented in
retinoblastoma, conjunctival melanoma, and choroidal melanoma[1-3]. 2. Latent
periods of up to thirty years have been observed in patients with choroidal
melanomas both prior to enucleation, and in the interval between enucleation
and development of metastatic disease[4-5]. 3. Approximately 65% of incompletely
excised basal cell carcinomas of the ocular adnexa do not recur[6].

There are a number of unresolved issues regarding the importance of immunologic factors in the host-tumor interaction. The biologic importance of

tumor-associated antigens in human malignancies is unknown. Do these antigens elicit a destructive response towards the tumor by the host's immune system, or are they biologically unimportant artifacts, and the measured immune reactivity towards them merely an epiphenomenon? Similarly, the relative importance of different components of the human host's immune system in the host-tumor interaction is unclear. In animal models, the importance of immune response genes, and various subsets of T-cells, B-cells, null cells, NK cells, and macrophages have been studied[7-11]. This type of data has not been well delineated in most human neoplasms.

Immunologic investigations of patients with ocular tumors could yield important information in four areas: 1. Immunologic tests could increase our ability to correctly differentiate primary ocular tumors from simulating lesions. 2. Immunologic tests could increase our ability to predict which patients with localized ocular neoplasms will develop widespread metastases. 3. Ocular malignancies may be a useful model to increase our understanding of immunologic mechanisms in human tumors. 4. An increased understanding of the importance of immunologic parameters in ocular malignancies may allow us to develop a rational basis for the potential use of immunotherapy in ocular tumors.

There are a number of advantages and disadvantages in the study of ocular neoplasms as a model of human tumor immunology. The advantages of this system include: 1. As previously described, ocular tumors have a high rate to spontaneous regressions consistent with the hypothesis that immunologic factors may be important. 2. In both choroidal melanoma and retinoblastoma the tumor mass can be detected at a much smaller size (and probably an earlier stage in their life cycle) than most other systemic malignancies. 3. The metastatic pattern of these ocular neoplasms is more homogenous than most systemic tumors.

There are a number of significant disadvantages in the study of ocular tumor immunology. 1. It is possible that these tumors arise in a "partially immunologically privileged site"[12]. 2. There is a paucity of available tumor tissue available for the purification of tumor-associated antigens. 3. There is an absence of relevant animal models of ocular malignancies. The striking exception to this point is the occurrence of the bovine squamous cell carcinoma model which has been useful in immunotherapy, however there are no adequate syngeneic models of choroidal melanoma, retinoblastoma, or orbital tumors.[13]

Most immunologic investigations of ocular tumors have been performed in humans. The status of these human investigations is reviewed below.

OCULAR MELANOMA IMMUNOLOGIC STUDIES

In choroidal melanoma patients non-specific and specific immunologic reactivity has been studied. Patients with primary choroidal melanomas do not
have significant alterations in non-specific cell-mediated immune status as
measured by either active or total rosettes, or by lymphocyte stimulation
with various mitogens[14-15]. Patients with metastatic choroidal melanoma have
alterations in non-specific cell-mediated immunologic status (decreased lymphocyte stimulation and rosette values), and elevated immune complex
levels[14-15]. Too few patients have been serially examined to determine the
prognostic sensitivity and specificity of non-specific cell-mediated immunologic assays however.

Choroidal melanoma patients have been demonstrated to have both cellular
and humoral immunologic reactivity towards melanoma-associated antigens. Anti-
melanoma antibodies have been observed in choroidal melanoma patients using
immunofluorescent techniques, however a significant number of false positive
results have occurred[16-18]. We and others have observed that as many as 50%
of patients will have false positive results when studied by immunofluorescent techniques[19-20]. In a study by Brownstein et al, 16 of 67 patients with
benign nevi and 15 of 56 controls have anti-melanoma antibodies[21]. Similarly,
Felberg and Federman observed a 24% incidence of anti-melanoma antibodies in
normal controls and 79% incidence in patients with metastatic choroidal
tumors[22]. Probably much of these data on specific humoral immunity towards
melanoma-associated antigens in choroidal melanoma patients is invalid. Recent studies by Old and his co-workers have demonstrated that at least three
distinct melanoma surface antigens are present on tumor cells. Rigid cross
testing must be performed to avoid the measurement of artifactitious reactivity towards either extraneous antigens or cross reactive normal tissue-associated antigens[23-25]. These controls have not been applied in the ocular
studies described above. These assays do not appear to have sufficient specificity for diagnostic use, however it is conceivable that they may be useful
prognostically. In one study a possible correlation between antibody levels
and response to photocoagulation in choroidal melanoma patients was observed,
however base line controls were not sufficiently rigid to draw definitive conclusions[26].

We have previously demonstrated cutaneous delayed hypersensitivity towards tumor-associated antigens in a number of human malignancies; in some reactivity has correlated with both disease status and prognosis[27].

Cutaneous delayed hypersensitivity towards melanoma-associated antigens
was studied in choroidal melanoma patients and subjects with simulating

lesions. Melanoma tissue was sterilely obtained from allogeneic tumor, processed by crude membrane extraction, gel chromatography, and continuous poly-
acrylamide-gel electrophoresis. This partially purified melanoma-associated
antigen was used to skin test a large group of subjects. Approximately 90%
of patients with pathologically confirmed choroidal melanomas had positive
skin test responses. In contrast, 4 of 27 patients with simulating lesions
had positive reaction[28]. There are two possible reasons for the false
positive skin test reaction which were observed: 1. The definition of a
positive skin test (> 6 mm of induration at 48 hours) is quantitative, not
qualitative, and based upon the desire to clinical discrimination between the
melanoma and control group. On biopsy of clinically negative standard recall
antigens skin test we have also observed histologic evidence of delayed hypersensitivity (unpathological observation). 2. Melanoma cells have both normal
and tumor-associated antigens. It is conceivable that the extraction and
purification techniques used, while enhancing for melanoma-associated antigens,
may not entirely eliminate tissue-associated antigens which could be responsible for the false positive responses.

While there is a marked statistically significant difference in skin
test reactivity between the choroidal melanoma and the simulating lesion
groups, the incidence of false positive reactivity precludes the use of skin
test assay diagnostically. There is insufficient data to determine whether
skin test reactivity will correlate with prognosis, and additional studies
must be performed.

We and others have demonstrated   in vitro cellular reactivity towards
melanoma-associated antigens using three molar KCl melanoma extracts in leukocyte migration inhibition type assays. In our laboratory we have observed
that certain melanoma-associated antigen preparations resulted in excellent
delineation between melanoma and control patients while other preparations
do not[29]. Presently this technique is not reliable enough for clinical diagnostic use since the specificity and sensitivity vary with different allogeneic
3 M KCl extracts and the same allogeneic material extracted by different
techniques (unpublished data).

Circulating immune complexes have been demonstrated in patients with a
number of human neoplasms[30]. We have begun serial studies on patients who
have been enucleated with high-risk choroidal melanoma. In one patient who
has developed metastatic choroidal melanoma, elevations of immune complex
levels were observed[31]. Further studies must be performed to determine
whether immune complex studies will be a sensitive prognostic adjunct.

IMMUNOLOGIC STUDIES IN RETINOBLASTOMA

Cell-mediated immunologic reactivity towards retinoblastoma-associated antigens have been demonstrated by some laboratories while other investigators have noted no significant differences[32-34]. The nature of the measured reactivity is unclear. It is doubtful that this activity is either towards HLA or virally-induced antigens; most likely the reactivity is towards tumor associated antigens shared by both retinoblastoma and normal retinal tissue[35].

Immune complexes have been demonstrated in a number of retinoblastoma patients[36]. While levels of circulating immune complexes have correlated with disease status and prognosis in some human malignancies, we have not studied a sufficient number of patients to determine if this is the case in retinoblastoma. We have performed preliminary characterization of the immune complexes from retinoblastoma sera using molecular sieve chromatography, affinity chromatography, and SDS-polyacrylamide gel electrophoresis (unpublished observations). Retinoblastoma patients' sera have two well defined peaks of immune complex activity on characterization with molecular sieve chromatography. These protein fractions had a molecular weight of approximately 1.6×10^5 daltons and 2.0×10^6 daltons.

Affinity chromatography with Sepharose 4B-Protein A and analytical polyacrylamide gel electrophoresis demonstrated that IgG was the predominate immunoglobulin in these complexes. On the basis of Sepharose-Concanavalin A affinity chromatography the antigen component of these complexes is a glycoprotein. Further studies to characterize the nature of the retinoblastoma-associated antigen are ongoing.

The detection of elevated levels of immune complexes in patients with retinoblastoma has at least three potential clinical applications: 1. This assay may be useful as diagnostic adjunct. 2. Levels of immune complexes may correlate with disease status and be useful prognostically. 3. Immune complex characterization may increase our ability to delineate the nature of retinoblastoma-associated antigens.

IMMUNOLOGIC STUDIES IN METASTATIC CHOROIDAL AND ADINEXA TUMORS

Immunologic alterations have been demonstrated in patients with metastatic ocular tumors. Approximately 50% of patients with metastatic tumors to choroid present to the Ophthalmologist prior to the discovery of the primary neoplasm[37]. In this clinical setting immunodiagnostic assays are potentially useful. Michaelson et al have demonstrated that approximately 50% of patients with metastatic choroidal tumors have CEA levels above 10 ug/ml; in contrast almost all primary choroidal melanoma patients have CEA levels below this value[38]. We have demonstrated that 91% of patients with metastatic chor-

oidal lesions have an elevated immune complex of CEA level, and when used
jointly these assays may be useful to differentiate primary from secondary
choroidal neoplasma[31]. Similarly, patients with metastatic lesions, especially if they are widespread, will often have alterations in non-specific
cell-mediated immunologic assays[39].

IMMUNOLOGIC STUDIES IN ORBITAL DISEASE

Approximately 20% of patients with orbital tumefaction have either
orbital lymphoma or orbital pseudotumor[40]. As many as 50% of these cases are
misdiagnosed using standard histologic techniques[41]. Applying lymphocyte
surface marker immunohistologic techniques to the study of orbital tumors, a
number of groups including our own have demonstrated that these studies hold
promise for improving our ability to clinically differentiate pseudotumor
from orbital lymphoma[42-44]. The specificity and sensitivity of these immunohistologic techniques in the differentiation of orbital neoplasms remains to
be determined.

CONCLUSIONS

Current understanding of the biologic importance of immunologic alterations in the human host-tumor is limited. In many human malignancies exis-
tance of tumor-associated antigens and host immunologic responses to them
have been demonstrated, however significant non-specific reactivity has also
been observed. More work must be performed to determine whether the reactivity towards these histologically specific human tumor-associated antigens is
important in the pathophysiology of malignancies or is an epiphenomenon.

Many of the tumor-associated antigens to which human reactivity has been
demonstrated may be tissue-associated, fetal, or viral antigens; further investigations on the nature of these tumor-associated antigens and ocular malignancies must be performed.

In most ocular malignancies, with the notable exception of orbital pseudotumor and orbital lymphoma, the diagnostic accuracy in ocular oncology units
is greater than 98%. Most likely, the major clinical application of these
experimental immunologic assays will be to increase our prognostic ability
and delineate those patients who will develop widespread metastatic disease.
This is especially important given the recent clinical trend to "conserva-
tively manage" patients with ocular tumors.

ACKNOWLEDGEMENTS

Supported in part by NIH Grants EY 1441, EY 1759 and EY 2072. Dr Char
is a recipient of an NIH Research Career Development Award (K04 EY117).

REFERENCES

1. Jensen, A.O., Anderson, S.R.: Spontaneous Regression of a Malignant Melanoma of the Choroid, Acta Ophthalmol. 52:173, 1974.

2. Khodadoust, A.A., Roozitalab, H.M., Smith, R.E., Green, W.R.: Spontaneous Regressions of Retinoblastoma. Surv. Ophthalmol. 21:467, 1977.

3. Reese, A.B.: Precancerous and Cancerous Melanosis. Am. J. Ophthalmol. 61:1272, 1966.

4. Newton, F.H.: Malignant Melanoma of Choroid. Arch. Ophthalmol. 73:198, 1965.

5. Duke-Elder, S.: System of Ophthalmology. Vol. 9, p. 872, 1966. C.V. Mosby, St. Louis.

6. Gooding, C.A., White, G., Yatsuchashi, M.: Significance of Marginal Extension in Excised Basal-cell Carcinoma. N. Engl. J. Med. 273:923, 1965.

7. Cantor, H., Shen, F.W., Boyse, E.A.: Separation of Helper T Cells from Suppressor T Cells Expressing Different Ly Components. II. Activation by Antigen: After Immunization, Antigen-specific Suppressor and Helper Activities are Mediated by Distinct T-Cell subclasses. J. Exp. Med. 143:1391, 1976.

8. Oehler, J.R., Herberman, R.B., Campbell, D.A., Jr., Djeu, J.Y.: Inhibition of Rat Mix Lymphocyte Cultures by Suppressor Macrophages. Cell. Immunol. 29:238-250, 1977.

9. Cooperband, S.R., Nimberg, R., Schmid, K., Mannick, J.A.: Humoral Immunosuppressive Factors. Transplant. Proc. 8:225-42, 1976.

10. Broder, S., Waldmann, T.A.: The Suppressor-Cell Network in Cancer. N. Engl. J. Med. 299:1335, 1978.

11. Old, L.J., Stockert, E., Boyse, E.A., Kim, J.H.: Antigenic Modulation. J. Exp. Med. 127:523, 1968.

12. Char, D.H.: Immunology of Uveitis and Ocular Tumors, Grune & Stratton, New York, New York, 1978.

13. Kleinschuster, S.J., Rapp, H.J., Lucker, D.C., Kainer, R.A.: Regression of Bovine Ocular Carcinoma by Treatment with a Myocobacterial Vaccine. J. Natl. Cancer Inst. 58:1807, 1977.

14. Char, D.H.: Immunologic Tests in Uveitis in Immunology and Immunopathology of the Eye. Silverstein, A.M. & O'Connor, G.R., eds., Masson, New York, 1979.

15. Priluk, J.A., Robertson, D.M., Pritchard, D.J.: Immune Profile in Choroidal Malignant Melanoma Patients. ARVO Meeting, May, 1978.

16. Rahi, A.H.S.: Autoimmune Reactions in Uveal Melanoma. Br. J. Ophthalmol. 55:793, 1971.

17. Wong, J.G., Oskvig, R.M.: Immunofluorescent Detection of Antibodies to Ocular Melanoma. Arch. Ophthalmol. 92:98, 1974.

18. Federman, J.L., Lewis, M.G., Clark, W.H.: Tumor-associated Antibodies to Ocular and Cutaneous Malignant Melanomas: Negative Interaction with Normal Choroidal Melanocytes. J. Natl. Cancer Inst. 52:587, 1974.

19. Whitehead, R.H.: Fluorescent Antibody Studies in Malignant Melanoma. Br. J. Cancer 28:525, 1973.

20. Wood. G.W., Barth, R.F.: Immunofluorescent Studies of Serologic Reactivity of Patients with Malignant Melanoma against Tumor-associated Cytoplasmic Antignes. J. Natl. Cancer Inst. 53:309, 1974.

21. Brownstein, S.,Sheikh, K.M., Lewis, M.G.: Immunological Studies in Patients with Malignant Melanoma of the Uvea. Can J. Ophthalmol. 12:16, 1977.

22. Felberg, N.T., Federman, J.L.: Tumor-associated Antibodies in Patients with Uveal Malignant Melanomas. ARVO 1978.

23. Carey, T.E., Takahashi, T., Resnick, L.A., Oettgen, H.F., Old, L.J.: Cell Surface Antigens of Human Malignant Melanoma: Mixed Hemadsorption Assays for Humoral Immunity to Cultures Autologous Melanoma Cells. Proc. Natl. Acad. Sci. USA 73:3278, 1976.

24. Shiku, H., Takahaski, T., Oettgen. H.F., Old, L.J.: Cell Surface Antigens of Human Malignant Melanoma. II. Serological Typing with Immune Adherence Assays and Definition of Two New Surface Antigens. J. Exp. Med. 144:873,1976.

25. Shiku, A., Takahaski, T., Resnick, L.A., Oettgen, H.F., Old, L.J.: Cell Surface Antigens of Human Malignant Melanoma III Recognition of Autoantibodies with Unusual Characteristics. J. Exp. Med. 145:784, 1977.

26. Federman, J.L., Sarin, L.K., Shields, J.A., Felberg, N.T.: Tumor-associated Antibodies in the Serum of Ocular Melanoma Patients II. Variation in Antibody Level following Xenon Arc Photocoagulation. Arch. Ophthalmol. 97: 252, 1979.

27. Char, D.H., Lepourhiet, A., Leventhal, B.S., and Herberman, R.B.: Cutaneous Delayed Hypersensitivity Responses to Tumor Associated and Other Antigens in Acute Leukemia. Int. J. Cancer, 12:409-419, 1973.

28. Char, D.H., Hollinshead, A., Cogan, D.G., Ballintine, E., Hogan, M.J. and Herberman, R.B.: Cutaneous Delayed Hypersensitivity Reactions to Soluble Melanoma Antigen in Patients with Ocular Melanoma. New England Journal of Medicine 291:274-277, 1974.

29. Char, D.H.: Inhibition of Leukocyte Migration with Melanoma-associated Antigens in Choroidal Tumors. Invest. Ophthal. 16:176-179, 1977.

30. Heier, H.E., Landaas, T.O., Marton, P.F.: Circulating Immune Complexes and Prognosis in Human Malignant Lymphoma. A Prospective Study. 1979. Int. Cancer 23:292.

31. Char, D.H., Christensen, M.: Immune Complexes and Carcinoembryonic Antigens Levels in Metastatic Choroidal Tumors. Am. J. Ophthalmol. 1979 (in press)

32. Char, D.H., Herberman, R.B.: Cutaneous Hypersensitivity Responses of Patients with Retinoblastoma to Standard Recall Antigens and Crude Membrane Extracts of Retinoblastoma Tissue Culture Cells. Am. J. Ophthalmol. 78:40, 1974.

33. Char, D.H., Ellsworth, R. Rabson, A.S., et al: Cell-mediated Immunity to a Retinoblastoma Tissue Culture Line in Patients with Retinoblastoma. Am. J. Ophthalmol. 78:5, 1974.

34. Mosier, M.A., Sulit, H.L.: Specific and Nonspecific Cellular Cytotoxicity Among Retinoblastoma Patients. ARVO meeting, April, 1975.

35. Char, D.H., Bergsma, D., Rabson, A.S., Albert, D.M., Herberman, R.B.: Cell Mediated Immunity to Retinal Antigens in Patients with Pigmentary Retinal Degenerations. Invest. Ophth. 13:198-203, 1974.

36. Char, D.H., Christensen, M., Goldberg, L., and Stein, P.: Immune Complexes in Retinoblastoma. Am. J. Ophthalmol. 86:395-399, 1978.

37. Font, R.L., Ferry, A.P.: Carcinoma Metastatic to the Eye and Orbit, 1976. Cancer 38:1326.

38. Michelson, J.B., Felberg, N.A.J., Shields, J.A.: Metastatic Adenocarcinoma 1978. Am. J. Ophthalmol. 86:142.

39. Char, D.H.: Immunology of Ocular Malignant Melanomas. Trans. Ophthal. Soc. U.K. 97:389-393, 1977.

40. Henderson, J.W.: Orbital Tumors. W.B. Saunders Company, Philadelphia 1973, Pg. 598.

41. Jakobiec, F.A., McLean, I., Font, R.I.: Clinicopathologic Characteristics of Orbital Lymphoid Hyperplasia. Ophthalmol, 1979 86:948.

42. Mann, R.B., Jaffe, E.S., Berard, C.W.: Malignant Lymphomas - A Conceptual Understanding of Morphologic Diversity. Am. J. Pathol. 1979, 94:103.

43. Knowles, D.M., Jakobiec, F.A., Halper, J.P.: Immunologic Characterization of the Ocular Adenxal Lymphoid Neoplasms. Am. J. Ophthalmol. 1979, 87:603.

44. Char, D.H.: Orbital Tumor Diagnosis: Lymphoma Versus Pseudotumor. Trans. Pacific Coast O & O (in press).

Immunological aspects of orbital inflammatory pseudotumors

G.M.Bleeker, M.D.

The Netherlands Ophthalmic Research Institute

Of the approximately 150 cases of orbital disorders presented yearly at the Orbital Center of the University of Amsterdam about one fifth concern intra-orbital inflammatory tumors. In addition to a variability of etiology and in clinical behavior the pathological definition of these tumors is far from uniform. In fact, these inflammatory tumors consist of a spectrum ranging from a granulomatous reaction to a foreign body on the one hand, to malignant lymphoma on the other. In between, one finds a range of inflammatory processes, characterized by a more intensive lymphocytic infiltration, lymphoid hyperplasia, follicular proliferation, gradually approaching the malignant non-Hodgkins lymphomas as registered by Rappaport[1]. This picture is completed by paraprotein producing lymphocytes as in multiple myeloma, Waldenstrom's Macroglobulinemia and also by Wegener's Granulomatosis. Finally, the Tolosa-Hunt syndrome is nothing more than a pseudotumor in the cavernous sinus.

The variability of pathology and clinical behavior is mirrored in the response to therapy. The more granulomatous cells the lesion has, the better its response to steroid treatment. Lymphosarcoma needs radiation or chemotherapy while Wegener's granulomatosis requires a combination of steroid therapy and cyclophosphamide.

Medical treatment of inflammatory tumors would greatly benefit from a more precise definition of the lesion involved. Considering the sometimes aggressive reaction of these inflammatory processes to surgery, it would be better to identify those lesions susceptible to medical treatment before surgery.

In 1973, we added immunology to our diagnostic armamentarium. In addition to the usual hematological investigation, protein content, para-protein and immunofluorescence examination were added. Immunofluorescence examination of tumor tissue and of bone marrow were carried out to define the cytological situation. Cytoplasmatic immunoglobulins and the kappa/lamda- ratio of light chains were estimated and membrane fluorescence was used to define the T-cell/B-cell ratio. On the basis of these investi-gations it was found that monoclonal immunoglobulins are characteristic of the more malignant components of pseudotumor, while polyclonal lesions are more benign in nature. In the case of monoclonal immunoglobulin production, the kappa/lamda ratio will show deviation from the normal (70:30).

Multiple myeloma, for instance, is characterized by monoclonality of the plasma-cell lesions, as expressed in the globulin and kappa/lamda- ratio. If light chains are produced, Bence-Jones protein may be demonstrated in the urine. We have learned that the investigations should not be confined to blood and tumor tissue, but that bone marrow should be inspected as well. If all three of these examinations are positive, it may be concluded that a generalized process is involved, while a normal bone marrow result would indicate a more localized process.

In particular, with respect to non-Hodgkin lymphomas it is of importance to determine whether they concern T-cell lymphocytes, B-cell lymphocytes, or as is sometimes noted, a non-T, non-B cell population. Both types of lymphocytes can be identified easily by modern immunological techniques (E-rosettes and ANAE-specks for the T-cells and SIg and EA-rosette for the B-cells and EA rosettes and diffuse ANAE for histiocytes).

Aberrations of the normal composition of 70% T-cells, 15% B-cells, and

10-15% non-T, non-B-cells can be indicative of the presence of a non-Hodgkin lymphoma; in particular the non-T, non-B-cell proliferation has a more malignant character than does B-cell proliferation. Since non-B cell lymphoproliferations do not produce immunoglobulins, the usual identification of monoclonality is less evident, but cell-function testing may be helpful.

Diseases like Waldenstrom's macroglobulinemia and Wegener's granulomatosis can be readily identified if approached according to this scheme. It is of utmost priority that immunological investigation is made use of extensively in the conditions described above since histological determination is far from ideal and also far from uniform.

In summary, I would recommend that we immediately introduce the clinical use of immunological methodology in lymphoproliferative disease of the orbit (and elsewhere), both because it is badly needed and also because the means are currently available.

LITERATURE CITED

1. Rappaport, H., C. Bernard, J.J. Butler, R.F. Dorfman, R.J. Lukes, and L.B. Thomas. 1971. Report of the committee on histopathological criteria contributing to staging of Hodgkin's disease. Cancer Res. 31:1864.

Some thoughts on tumor immunology and immunotherapy

Osias Stutman

Cellular Immunobiology Section, Memorial Sloan-Kettering Cancer Center, New York, New York 10021

INTRODUCTION

The original title of my talk, as proposed by the organizers of this Workshop, was "Tumors as Graft Models; Value of Tumor Immunotherapy." I took the liberty of changing the title, because if not, this paper may have ended after two short statements: 1) spontaneous tumors are not graft models, and even transplanted tumors represent a very special type of graft (1, 2) and 2) immunotherapy is presently under a thorough re-examination with respect to its clinical value (3, 4).

TUMOR IMMUNOLOGY

Although a vast amount of study on the immunology of experimental tumors has been going on since the beginning of the century (see Woglom's review of 1929 with a few hundred references, 5), it was only in 1973 that "Tumor Immunology" was enthroned as a sub-section (separate from "Cellular Immunology") within the Journal of Immunology.

One of the distinct features of the immune response to tumors, as well as the immune response to many parasites (6), which is not observed in transplantation immunology, is the phenomenon of "concomitant immunity" (7). Although first observed by Paul Ehrlich in 1906 (8), the phenomenon was considered immunological by Bashford in 1908, who also coined the term (7). In essence, concomitant immunity is the observed resistance to a second tumor graft in animals with progressive growth of the primary tumor (7, 8). It took almost 60 years for this phenomenon to be re-discovered (2, 9). And most importantly, it still remains essentially unexplained, whatever the mechanisms proposed (10-13). Another evidence of such concomitant immunity was the adoptive transfer of immunity to naive hosts with lymphoid cells from the tumor-bearing animals (14-16), or the demonstration of in vitro immune responses to the tumors (17-20). The fact that concomitant immunity or some form of immune reactivity is detected in tumor bearing patients against their own tumors

(17-20), further stresses the importance of this phenomenon.

Another important step to establish tumor immunology as a reputable discipline was the unequivocal demonstration that experimentally-induced tumors in inbred animals were antigenic for the syngeneic hosts (15, 18, 21-27). References 21 and 22 are included because they represent a good example of poorly designed experiments that ended up being correct, when the proper experimental design was used (15, 23-25). The demonstration that spontaneously arising tumors in experimental animals are poorly immunogenic (28-30), as well as the difficulties in defining likely candidates for tumor-associated antigens in man (18, 31, 32), has cast some doubts on the validity of the induced-tumor models. However, the present day epidemiology of human cancer and the impact of man-made environmental factors, actually casts some doubts on the validity of some of the experimental models themselves.

The fact that many of the studies that defined the genetics of transplantation, as well as the development of inbred mouse strains, has used tumors as transplants (33-35), or that many of the in vitro assays to measure cell-mediated cytotoxicity after allo-sensitization use tumor cells as targets (20, 36), is probably behind the thought that tumors may represent a special type of "graft." As a matter of fact, one of the reasons that the initial studies in tumor immunity (5) fell into disrepute, was the demonstration of "false positive" rejections due to normal histocompatibility antigens in the non-inbred or partially inbred animals (37).

As was indicated above, in many experimental systems, tumor antigenicity may be difficult to demonstrate, and it is accepted that not all tumors (spontaneous or induced) may show detectable antigenicity when measured in vivo (28-30, 38, 39), although some of such tumors may show antigenicity in in vitro testing (as seems to be the case for mouse lung adenomas, 40). Burnet addressed this point as supportive of his immunosurveillance theory (41). However, tumors of low or undetectable antigenicity can appear regardless of the immunological status of the host (38, 39) and can even be detected in mice with life-long profound immunodepression (39, 42). In addition, tumors produced within cell-impermeable diffusion chambers which are not exposed to cellular immunity (44) can also show the whole spectrum of antigenicity, including tumors with low or undetectable antigenicity. The surveillance theory would have predicted that in the absence of immunoselection, strongly antigenic tumors would be expressed in excess (41). These discussions on tumor antigenicity or immunogenicity are highly pertinent if we adhere to the ideas that tumors are handled by the immune system in the same way as allografts and that such immune responses are highly specific and to

a large extent thymus-dependent (1, 2, 4, 9-20, 36, 41, 44). Whatever the
role applied to the immune system in defense against tumors (i.e. defense
against incipient tumor, in essence what is known as "immunological surveillance" as in 41; or reaction against an established tumor which represents
the domain of tumor immunology), the choice of the thymus-dependent system
as the exclusive executor of these responses is difficult to understand (for
critiques of immune surveillance and its thymus dependency, see 39, 42, 45,
46; for critiques of the thymus-dependency of tumor rejection, see 47-50).
One possible interpretation is the equation of such defense mechanism with
allograft rejection in which T cells play an important, albeit not an exclusive role (51). The other being, perhaps, the enthusiasm as a result of
the announcement of the "golden age of thymology" in 1967 (52). On the
other hand, it is surprising that the leads obtained form the studies on
cellular immunity to infectious or parasitic agents (53-56), were so slowly
applied to studies on tumor immunity.

Although cellular immunology has developed into a complex system of
precursor, effector, regulatory and amplifier compartments, which include
antigen specific and nonspecific steps, as well as a variety of soluble mediators and recruitment devises, we still ignore many of the fine details of
the system. Especially concerning local versus systemic activities. And it
is obvious, that such fine details are still almost totally undefined in
models in which an anti-tumor immune response is studied. I will draw from
our own work to demonstrate that even when the focus is concentrated only
on the T cell-mediated cytotoxic response, as we have done with a mouse mammary adenocarcinoma syngeneic model, we have found that complex T-T interactions regulate the response in the regional node, and that different subsets of effector cells are generated as a consequence of such response (57,
58). However, just to point to one single problem, the peak T cytotoxic
activity in the regional node appears rapidly and declines, while in vivo
transplantation immunity (i.e. the capacity to reject a transplanted tumor)
still remains for much longer periods of time (57, 59).

In addition, whatever our position concerning the role of T cells as
surveillance devices (42, 45, 46) or as effector cells in anti-tumor immunity
(57-59), other immune mechanisms have to be considered. Especially the
non-adoptive immunities which can be detected in normal individuals, without
prior stimulation. Such "natural" defense mechanisms include macrophages
(49, 53-56) and "natural killer" or similar mechanisms (50, 60-62). Both
cell types have been, indeed, proposed as mediators of some form of anti-
tumor surveillance (47, 48, 50, 60-63). I will not dwell on the fine details

of both systems, since there is an extensive bibliography on macrophage-mediated cytotoxicity or cytostasis of tumor cells (49, 56, 64-65) as well as on the recently defined natural killer (NK) cells (50, 60, 61) and natural cytotoxic (NC) cells (62). NK cells have been defined mostly against lymphoma targets in suspension (59, 60, 61) and NC cells against adherent targets derived from solid tumors (62). Although showing some minor differences, both systems share a substantial number of properties, especially the fact that the effector lymphoid cells do not have the characteristics of mature T, B or macrophages (50, 60-62, 66).

However, several aspects of these systems of "natural" responses should be noted: a) both mechanisms, macrophages and NK-NC cells have been described in animals as well as in man (20, 49, 50, 60, 61, 67); b) both have been considered as candidates for alternative (i.e. T-independent) antitumor surveillance (47, 48, 50, 61-67); c) both activated macrophages with antitumor cytotoxicity (66, 68), as well as NK-NC cells (59, 60-62) have been described in nude athymic mice, and have been considered responsible for the "normal" tumor incidence in such animals (42, 45, 56, 50); d) both systems are quite resistant to immunodepressive procedures that affect T or B cells, thus, any of the two mechanisms may still be exerting its putative surveillance functions in a variety of models which used immunodepression of the host as a tool to define the possible role of immune functions in tumor control (42, 45, 46, 50); e) the levels of activity in the NK system are apparently regulated by interferon (i.e. interferon as well as a variety of interferon inducers can augment NK activity, 69-71).

In addition, neither system apparently recognizes "tumor associated transplantation antigens" nor "tumor associated surface antigens" (18). The surface structures being recognized by macrophages and NK-NC cells are still undefined (49, 50, 60-67). Thus, the question of tumor antigenicity discussed previously, which was not important for the thymus-dependent tumor immunity (41, 47, 48), becomes trivial. Similarly, the problem of "lack of antigenicity" of most spontaneous tumors in experimental animals and man (38-33), also becomes of lesser import, since such tumors may still be susceptible to attack by either NK-NC cells or macrophages. As a matter of fact, one of the non-antigenic tumors described in ref. 30, showed a high susceptibility to _in vivo_ growth inhibition by C. parvum-activated macrophages (72). However, we cannot exclude interactions between the systems, as well as influence by the conventional immune responses. For example, the macrophage content in tumors induced by the Moloney sarcoma virus in nude mice was markedly reduced and correlated with absence of regression of such tumors

(73). This may suggest that macrophage mobilization and/or activation in this model may be regulated by a thymus-dependent mechanism.

It should be noted that the in vitro reactivity of lymphoid cells from normal individuals against tumor cells was described in 1973 (74), and probably observed by many investigators before that, but dismissed as trivial, due to the obsessive quest for "specific" anti-tumor responses (75). For further discussion on the use of the "normal control" data in in vitro cytotoxicity studies in animals and man, see ref. 20.

There is evidence that the NK system can handle in vivo small inocula of tumor cells (60). As we discussed in previous reviews (42, 45), a similar defense mechanism operated by specific T cells would, probably, be inoperative. For such a T cell mechanism to be operative, it would be necessary for the antigenic tumor to appear rapidly and in sufficient numbers to provoke a fully immunogenic stimulus. Anything less would either pass undetected or would result in an inefficient immune response against the emerging tumor (42, 45, 76), perhaps even stimulating tumor growth (77). Even in the case of microorganisms which are highly antigenic, it takes a relatively large antigenic stimulus to produce a specific T response that can be measured (54). In brucellosis, for example, the infection waxes and wanes because the immunogenic stimulus from a declining bacterial population permits resistance to decline and subsequently allows the parasite to grow until an antigenic stimulus is large enough to reactivate the host's immune response (54). If defense against an infectious agent demands such a strong antigenic stimulus, it seems unlikely that a small amount of transformed cells, would actually provoke a protective specific immune response, even assuming that such tumor cells have the strongest antigens. Thus, our criticism of the thymus-dependent tumor immunity or immune surveillance as true protective devices (42, 45, 46). Based on the in vitro and in vivo experimental data on the "natural" or non-specific (or perhaps "less-specific") responses, these criticisms do not apply, or at least do not appear as strong. If it is the dream of the cancer immunotherapist of some form of "immune" response seeking and destroying the remaining tumor cells after conventional therapy which reduces the tumor mass (3, 4), then it is most probable that the non-specific mechanisms discussed may be more effective than the specific ones. The fact that most human tumors studied appear as monoclonal (78), may argue against these natural defense mechanisms as being effective, since single or small numbers of cells have to pass undetected for the monoclonal tumor to arise. However, it may also be argued that monoclonality of the clinical tumor is the consequence of some in vivo selection and subsequent clonal dominance during tumor progression.

George and Eva Klein (46) pointed out "the central fallacy of tumor immunology" in 1977, which summarizes well our discussion of the subject. The fallacy includes the following aspects: all tumors are potentially recognized by the host immune response (i.e. the problem of antigenicity); tumor development is always a consequence of a breakdown of the response (i.e. the immune surveillance problem) and finally, therapy must "strive to correct the breakdown" (i.e. the problem of immunotherapy). Among the possible reasons for the development of the fallacy, one may cite: the surveillance concept in a generalized and dogmatic form (see critiques 42, 45); the pressures to achieve practical results (see 3, 4) or even "...biased evaluation with disregard for the widespread occurrence of nonselective cytotoxicity" (46). This last point is what we called the obsessive quest for "specific" antitumor responses in vitro. We will not repeat our stances against dogma, wishful thinking and uncritical generalizations in goal oriented research (42, 45), but an awareness of the problem is probably the main corrective step to avoid such behavior.

We ignore so many facets of the local and systemic events of an antitumor response mounted by a tumor-bearing individual, both in animals and man, that to project a special strategy for the study of ocular tumors appears naive.

Without going into details of how the immune reactions operate in the eye compartments, a few examples of different behavior of eye versus systemic tumors may be pertinent, even if used as examples of our lack of understanding of what is going on. Spontaneous remissions or regressions of choroidal melanomas have been described (79); melanomas of the choroid and conjunctiva can remain stationary for long time (80); 50% of the patients with choroidal metastases show ocular signs prior to discovery of the primary tumor (81). Are these examples telling us that special local conditions, whether immunological or not, may be crucial in determining tumor progression?

IMMUNOTHERAPY

Although there is a major trend for non-specific immunotherapy procedures (3, 4, 82-85), especially of the active type (i.e. by administration of immunostimulants to the tumor-bearing host), the ultimate goal of immunotherapy is the active specific form, for which "tumor anitgens" have to be defined (86).

At the risk of being repetitious, I will insist that our present stage of knowledge (or ignorance) about specific and non-specific antitumor immune responses, as well as the unsolved riddle of "concomitant immunity" or the

question of relevant or irrelevant tumor antigens, only permits some educated guessing concerning the mechanism of immunotherapy procedures. Thus,
immunotherapy remains essentially empirical.

Probably, the major problem that the immunotherapist is confronting is
overinterpretation of the results and the unconscious (hopefully) bias
towards success. The need of properly designed trials with concurrent controls (instead of historical controls) is so obvious that it will not be
discussed any further (3, 4).

In general, local non-specific active immunotherapy is more successful
than systemic administration (3, 4, 83, 84), and this aspect may have some
relevance to ocular tumors.

One interesting model under study is that of the bovine ocular squamous
carcinoma or "cancer eye" (87) and tumor regressions have been reported
after local administration of a Mycobacterial vaccine (88). However, this
study is a good example of bias and overinterpretation. For example, it is
quite clear that the evolution of the disease is quite different depending
on tumor location (87), thus, conjunctival tumors rarely metastasize, while
lid tumors have a high metastasis rate and poor prognosis. Thus, the disease has two very different clinical manifestations, depending on eye versus
lid tumors (87). However, in the therapy study, all the regressions were
observed in the "eye" group while no clear effect of the treatment was observed in the "lid"tumors (88). In addition, lid tumors were under-repre-
sented in the "experimental" versus the control groups, compounding the problem of design and evaluation of this study (88).

Only well designed experimental and clinical trials, even based on purely
empirical grounds, will generate some progress, no matter how avidly we
expect success.

CONCLUSIONS

There is no doubt that, once a substantial mass of tumor has developed
in the host, some form of specific immunity can be demonstrated. Whether
such specific immune responses (mediated by T cells or other mechanisms)
can be used as a potential immunotherapy device, is clearly the goal of
tumor immunology. However, the recently described "natural" cytotoxic
mechanisms, which may play a role in controlling incipient tumor development,
can be considered as alternative or complementary devises that can be used
for the immunological therapy of cancer.

However, it is also apparent that due to the highly emotional image
that cancer has in our present day society (89), a remarkable voluntarism
has developed in the scientific community, which has, in some instances, dul-

led the scientific perception of the actual problems represented by the tumor-bearing individual.

REFERENCES

1. Amos, D.B. 1962. The use of simplified systems as an aid to the interpretation of mechanisms of graft rejection. Progr. Allergy 6: 468.
2. Mikulska, Z.B., C. Smith and P. Alexander. 1966. Evidence for an immunological reaction of the host directed against its own actively growing primary tumor. J. Natl. Cancer Inst. 36: 29.
3. Terry, W.D. and D. Windhorst (eds.) 1977. Immunotherapy of Cancer: Present Status of Trials in Man. Raven Press, New York.
4. Southam, C.M. and Friedman, H. (eds.). 1976. International Conference on Immunotherapy of Cancer. Ann. N.Y. Acad. Sci. 277.
5. Woglom, W.H. 1929. Immunity to transplantable tumors. Cancer Rev. 4: 129.
6. Bloom, B.R. 1979. Games parasites play: How parasites evade immune surveillance. Nature 279: 21.
7. Bashford, E.F., J.A. Murray, M. Haaland and W.H. Bowen. 1908. General results of propagation of malignant new growths. Third Sci. Rep. Imperial Cancer Res. Fund. London. 3: 262.
8. Ehrlich, P. 1906. Experimentelle Karzinomstudien an Mausen. Arb. Inst. Exp. Ther. Frankfurt. 1: 65.
9. Gershon, R.K., R.L. Carter and K. Knodo. 1967. On concomitant immunity in tumor-bearing hamsters. Nature 213: 674.
10. Hellstrom, I., K.E. Hellstrom and H.O. Sjogren. 1970. Serum mediated inhibition of cellular immunity to methylcholanthrene-induced murine sarcomas. Cell Immunol. 1: 18.
11. Youn, J.K., D. LeFrancois and G. Barski. 1973. In vitro studies on mechanism of the "eclipse" of cell-mediated immunity in mice bearing advanced tumors. J. Natl. Cancer Inst. 50: 921.
12. Vaage, J. 1973. Concomitant immunity and specific desensitization in murine tumor hosts. Israel J. Med. Sci. 9: 332.
13. Friedman, H. and C. Southam (eds.). 1976. International Conference of Immunobiology of Cancer. Ann. N.Y. Acad. Sci. 276.
14. Mitchison, N.A. 1954. Passive transfer of transplantation immunity. Proc. Roy. Soc. (Biol.) 142: 72.
15. Old, L.J., E.A. Boyse, D.A. Clarke and E. Carswell. 1962. Antigenic properties of chemically induced tumors. Ann. N.Y. Acad. Sci. 101: 80.
16. Bard, D.S., W.G. Hammond and Y.H. Pilch. 1969. The role of the regional lymph nodes in the immunity to a chemically induced sarcoma in C3H mice. Cancer Res. 29: 1379.
17. Klein, G. 1971. Immunological studies on a human tumor. Dilemmas of the experimentalist. Isr. J. Med. Sci. 7: 111.
18. Herberman, R.B. 1977. Immunogenicity of tumor antigens. Biochim. Biophys. Acta 473: 93.
19. Herberman, R.B. 1977. Existence of Tumor Immunity in Man IN Mechanisms of Tumor Immunity. Green, I., S. Cohen and R.T. McCluskey, eds. J. Wiley & Sons. New York, p. 175.
20. Bloom, B.R. and J.R. David (eds.) 1976. In Vitro Methods in Cell-mediated and Tumor Immunity. Academic Press, New York.
21. Gross, L. 1943. Intradermal immunization of C3H mice against a sarcoma that originated in an animal of the same line. Cancer Res. 3: 326.
22. Foley, E.J. 1953. Antigenic properties of methylcholanthrene-induced tumors in mice of the strain of origin. Cancer Res. 13: 835.
23. Prehn, R.T. and J.M. Main. 1957. Immunity to methylcholanthrene-induced sarcomas. J. Natl. Cancer Inst. 18: 769.

24. Klein, G., H.O. Sjogren, E. Klein and K.E. Hellstrom. 1960. Demonstration of resistance against methylcholanthrene-induced sarcomas in the primary autochtonous host. Cancer Res. 20: 1561.

25. Sjogren, H.O. 1961. Further studies on the induced resistance against isotransplantation of polyoma tumors. Virology 15: 214.

26. Old, L.J. and E.A. Boyse. 1964. Immunology of experimental tumors. Ann. Rev. Med. 15: 167.

27. Klein, G. 1968. Tumor-specific transplantation antigens. Cancer Res. 28: 625.

28. Baldwin, R.W. 1966. Tumor-specific immunity against spontaneous rat tumors. Int. J. Cancer 1: 257.

29. Prehn, R.T. 1969. The relationship of immunology to carcinogenesis. Ann. N.Y. Acad. Sci. 164: 449.

30. Hewitt, H.B., E.R. Blake and A.S. Walder. 1976. A critique of the evidence for active host defense against cancer based on personal studies of 27 murine tumours of spontaneous origin. Br. J. Cancer 33: 241.

31. Klein, G. 1975. Immunological surveillance against neoplasia. Harvey Lectures 69: 71.

32. Shiku, H., T. Takahashi, H.F. Oettgen and L.J. Old. 1976. Cell surface antigens of human malignant melanoma. II. Serological typing with immune adherence assays and definition of two new surface antigens. J. Exp. Med. 144: 873.

33. Little, C.C. and E.E. Tyzzer. 1916. Further experimental studies on the inheritance of susceptibility to a transplantable tumor, carcinoma (JWA) of the Japanese waltzing mouse. J. Med. Res. 33: 393.

34. Corer, P.A. 1937. The genetic and antigenic basis of tumor transplantation. J. Pathol. Bacteriol. 44: 691.

35. Snell, G.D. 1953. The genetics of transplantation. J. Natl. Cancer Inst. 14: 691.

36. Henney, C.S. 1977. T-cell-mediated cytolysis: An overview of some current issues. Contemp. Top. Immunobiol. 7: 245.

37. Eisen, M.J. and W.H. Woglom. 1941. The non-specific nature of induced resistance to tumors. Cancer Res. 1: 629.

38. Bartlett, G.L. 1972. Effect of host immunity on the antigenic strength of primary tumors. J. Natl. Cancer Inst. 49: 493.

39. Stutman, O. 1972. Immunologic studies on resistance to oncogenic agents in mice. Natl. Cancer Inst. Monogr. 35: 107.

40. Colnaghi, M.I., D. Menard and G. Della Porta. 1971. Demonstration of cellular immunity against urethan-induced lung adenomas in mice. J. Natl. Cancer Inst. 47: 1325.

41. Burnet, F.M. 1971. Immunologic surveillance in neoplasia. Transplant. Rev. 7: 3.

42. Stutman, O. 1975. Immunodepression and malignancy. Adv. Cancer Res. 22: 261.

43. Mondal, S., P.T. Iype, L.M. Griesbach and C. Heidelberger. 1970. Antigenicity of cells derived from mouse prostate after malignant transformation in vitro by carcinogenic hydrocarbons. Cancer Res. 30: 1593.

44. Parmiani, G., C. Carbone and R.T. Prehn. 1972. In vivo and in vitro methylcholanthrene carcinogenesis in diffusion chambers. Tumori 58: 326.

45. Stutman, O. 1977. Immunological surveillance, IN Origins of Human Cancer. Hiatt, H.H., J.D. Watson and J.W. Winsten (eds.). Cold Spring Harbor Lab., Cold Spring, N.Y. p. 729.

46. Stutman, O. 1978. Spontaneous, viral and chemically induced tumors in the nude mouse, IN The Nude Mouse in Experimental and Clinical Research. Fogh, J. and B. Giovanella (eds.). Academic Press, New York. p. 411.

47. Klein, G. and E. Klein. 1977. Rejectability of virus-induced tumors and nonrejectability of spontaneous tumors: A lesson in contrasts. Transplant. Proc. 9: 1095.

48. Klein, G. and E. Klein. 1977. Immune surveillance against virus-induced tumors and nonrejectability of spontaneous tumors: Contrasting consequences of host versus tumor evolution. Proc. Natl. Acad. Sci. USA 74:2121.

49. Alexander, P. 1976. The functions of the macrophage in malignant disease. Ann. Rev. Med. 27: 207.

50. Herberman, R.B. and H.T. Holden. 1978. Natural cell-mediated immunity. Adv. Cancer Res. 27: 305.

51. Russell, P.S. and A.B. Cosimi. 1979. Transplantation. New Eng. J. Med. 301: 470.

52. Miller, J.F.A.P. 1967. The thymus. Yesterday, today and tomorrow. Lancet II: 1299.

53. Mackaness, G.B. and R.V. Blanden. 1967. Cellular Immunity. Progr. Allergy 11: 89.

54. Mackaness, G.B. 1969. The influence of immunologically committed lymphocytes in macrophage activity in vivo. J. Exp. Med. 129: 973.

55. Nelson, D.S. 1974. Immunity to infection, allograft immunity and tumor immunity: Parallels and contrasts. Transplant. Rev. 19: 226.

56. Mackaness, G.B. 1976. Role of macrophages in host defense mechanisms. IN The Macrophage in Neoplasia. Fink , M.A. (ed.) Academic Press, New York, p. 3.

57. Stutman, O., F.W. Shen and E.A. Boyse. 1977. Ly phenotype of T cells cytotoxic for syngeneic mouse mammary tumors: evidence for T cell interactions. Proc. Natl. Acad. Sci. USA 74: 5667.

58. Stutman, O. and F.W. Shen 1978. H2 restriction and non-restriction of T cell mediated cytotoxicity against mouse mammary tumor targets. Nature 276: 181.

59. Stutman, O. 1976. Correlation of in vivo and in vitro studies of antigens relevant to control of murine breast cancer. Cancer Res. 36: 737.

60. Kiessling, R. and O. Haller. 1978. Natural killer cells in the mouse: An alternative surveillance mechanism? Contemp. Top. Immunobiol. 8: 171.

61. Moller, G. (ed.) 1979. Natural Killer Cells. Immunological Rev. 44.

62. Stutman, O., C.J. Paige, and E. Feo Figarella. 1978. Natural cytotoxic cells against solid tumors in mice. I. Strain and age distribution and target cell susceptibility. J. Immunol. 121: 1819.

63. Alexander, P. 1976. Surveillance against neoplastic cells- Is it mediated by macrophages? Br. J. Cancer 33: 344.

64. Hibbs, Jr., J.B., H.A. Chapman, Jr. and J.B. Einberg. 1978. The macrophage as antineoplastic surveillance cell: biological perspectives. J. Reticuloendothel. Soc. 24: 549.

65. Keller, R. 1976. Susceptibility of normal and transformed lines to cytostatic and cytotoxic effects of macrophages. J. Natl. Cancer Inst. 56: 369.

66. Paige, C., E. Feo Figarella, M.J. Cuttito, A. Cahan and O. Stutman. 1978. Natural cytotoxic cells against solid tumors in mice. II. Some characteristics of the effector cells. J. Immunol. 121: 1827.

67. Pross, H.F. and M.G. Baines. 1977. Spontaneous human lymphocyte-mediated cytotoxicity against tumor target cells. VI. A brief review. Cancer Immunol. Immunother. 3: 75.

68. Meltzer, M.S. 1976. Tumoricidal responses in vitro of peritoneal macrophages from conventionally housed and germfree nude mice. Cell. Immunol. 22: 176.

69. Trinchieri, G., D. Santoli and H. Koprowski. 1978. Spontaneous cell-mediated cytotoxicity in humans. Role of interferon and immunoglobulins. J. Immunol. 120: 1849.

70. Gidlund, M., A Orn, H. Wigzell, A. Senik and I. Gresser. 1978. Enhanced NK cell activity in mice injected with interferon and interferon inducers. Nature 273: 759.

71. Djeu, J.Y., J.A. Heinbaugh, H.T. Holden and R.B. Herberman. 1979. Augmentation of mouse natural killer cell activity by interferon and interferon inducers. J. Immunol. 122: 175.

72. Woodruff, M.F.A., V.L. Whitehead and G. Speedy. 1978. Studies with a spontaneous mouse tumor. I. Growth in normal mice and response to Corynebacterium Parvum. Br. J. Cancer 37: 345.

73. Stutman, O. 1975. Delayed tumor appearance and absence of regression in nude mice infected with murine sarcoma virus. Nature 253: 142.

74. Takasugi, M., M.R. Mickey and P.I. Terasaki. 1973. Reactivity of lymphocytes from normal persons on cultured tumor cells. Cancer Res. 33: 2898.

75. Hellstrom, K.E. and I. Hellstrom. 1974. Lymphocyte-mediated cytotoxicity and blocking serum activity to tumor antigens. Adv. Immunol. 18: 209.

76. Andrews, E.J. 1974. Failure of immunosurveillance against chemically induced in situ stumors. J. Natl. Cancer Inst. 52: 729.

77. Prehn, R.T. 1972. The immune reaction as stimulator of tumor growth. Science 176: 70.

78. Friedman, J.M. and P.J. Fialkow. 1976. Cell marker studies of human tumorigenesis. Transplant. Rev. 28: 17.

79. Jensen, O.A. and S.R. Andersen. 1974. Spontaneous regression of a malignant melanoma of the choroid. Acta Ophtalmol. 52: 173.

80. Newton, F.H. 1965. Malignant melanoma of the choroid. Arch. Ophtalmol. 73: 198.

81. Ferry, A.P. 1973. Biologic behavior and pathologic features of carcinoma metastatic to the eye and orbit. Amer. Ophtalmol. Soc. Trans. 71:372.

82. Currie, G.A. 1972. Eighty years of immunotherapy: A review of immunological methods used for the treatment of human cancer. Br. J. Cancer 26: 141.

83. Bast Jr., R.C., B.S. Bast and H.J. Rapp. 1976. Critical review of previously reported animal studies of tumor immunotherapy with non-specific immuno-stimulants. Ann. N.Y. Acad. Sci. 277: 60.

84. Mastrangelo, M.J., D. Berd and R.E. Bellet. 1976. Critical review of previously reported clinical trials of cancer immunotherapy with non-specific immunostimulants. Ann. N.Y. Acad. Sci. 277: 94.

85. Murphy, S. and E. Hersh. 1978. Immunotherapy of leukemia and lymphoma. Sem. Hematol. 15: 181.

86. Oettgen, H.F. 1977. Immunotherapy of cancer. New Eng. J. Med. 297: 484.

87. Russell, W.O., E.S. Wynne and G.S. Loquvam. 1956. Studies on bovine ocular squamous carconoma ("Cancer Eye"). Cancer 9: 1.

88. Kleinschuster, S.J., H.J. Rapp, D.C. Leuker and R.A. Kainer. 1977. Regression of bovine ocular carcinoma by treatment with a mycobacterial vaccine. J. Natl. Cancer Inst. 58: 1807.

89. Sontag, S. 1978. Illness as Metaphor. Farrar, Strauss and Giroux, New York.

Immunobiology of the cornea

Arthur M.Silverstein

The Johns Hopkins University School of Medicine, Baltimore, Maryland

ABSTRACT

The usual avascularity of the cornea, and certain features of its structure, confer on corneal grafts a degree of immuno-logical privilege. This may take the form of interruption of the afferent arc of sensitization and/or the efferent arc of graft rejection. However, corneal grafts may undergo rejection under certain circumstances. This review examines the various factors responsible for both privilege and rejection, and emphasizes the advantages possessed by experimental corneal models for the study of basic mechanisms of allograft rejection.

INTRODUCTION

The ability of the corneal graft to maintain clarity in the recipient eye makes keratoplasty almost unique in the field of clinical tissue and organ transplantation. The elegant demon-strations by Medawar[1,2] and by Billingham et al.[3] that allograft rejection is based upon specific immunologic reaction to histoincompatible antigens of the donor led to the early conclusion that the corneal graft must be exempt from histo-incompatibility and other immunologic considerations. It was because of the frequent success of the keratoplasty procedure, and also because of the difficulty of diagnosing immunologic rejection of the cornea, that those instances of corneal graft failure that were observed were usually attributed to a variety of non-immunologic causes.[4,5]

A number of explanations were advanced to explain the basis for the exemption from immunologic rejection enjoyed by the corneal graft. These included: 1) the absence of appropriate antigens on the cellular elements of the cornea; 2) the rapid death of donor cellular elements and their replacement by the host before they could stimulate an active immune response; 3) an "adaptation" of the graft within the recipient cornea, causing it thenceforth to be insusceptible to specific rejection even in the actively sensitized host; and 4) the existence of a special privilege conferred upon the graft by virtue of unique characteristics of the corneal site itself. But it was soon demonstrated by Paufique et al.[6] and in the careful investigations by Maumenee[7-9] that the corneal graft might indeed be subject to immunologic rejection, and that this process probably accounts for a substantial proportion of late failures of corneal allografts. These observations prompted numerous investigators to reexamine each of the factors which might contribute to immunologic privilege where it exists, and to specific graft rejection when it occurs. In this review, we will reexamine the most pertinent details of such studies, so that the phenomenology of the transplantation and rejection of corneal allografts may be reasonably compared with that of other solid tissues.

THE STRUCTURE OF THE CORNEA

The cornea is structurally a fairly simple tissue, whose principal physiologic function is to maintain transparency along the visual axis. It is composed of three layers (Fig. 1) - a stratified epithelium adjacent to the tear film, which lies upon a basement membrane; a stroma, composed of a highly organized and transparent collagenous lattice, sparsely populated by keratocytes; and an endothelium consisting of a monolayer of

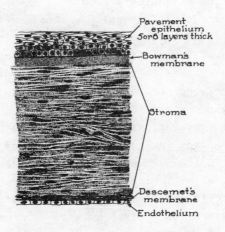

Figure 1. The structure of the normal cornea.

cells distributed in a highly uniform pattern on a very thick
Descemet's membrane.

The epithelial layer not only provides protection against
exogenous pathogens, but also contributes somewhat to the
maintenance of corneal clarity. However, it is characterized by
the ability to heal even large epithelial defects with great
rapidity, by a process of epithelial sliding and mitosis, so
that a corneal graft from which the epithelium has been removed
will very rapidly be recovered by host epithelium, and this is a
procedure frequently used clinically with impunity.

The corneal stroma is somewhat unique in that it will
maintain crystal clarity even when its keratocytes are dead. It
is for this reason that a lamellar (partial thickness lacking
endothelium) corneal graft of even lyophilized stroma will provide
a satisfactorily clear result.

It is the corneal endothelium which is physiologically the
most important and critical element for transplantation purposes.
The principal function of the endothelium is the physiologic
maintenance of corneal clarity, so that when the endothelium is
compromised the cornea will become cloudy, leading to edema and
neovascularization which may set the stage for sensitization by
and rejection of the penetrating (full thickness) corneal graft.
In the human, the corneal endothelium heals only very slowly if
at all, so that destruction of the endothelium of a corneal graft
almost assures graft failure. It is this critical role of the
corneal endothelium that renders the penetrating graft much more
susceptible to rejection than the lamellar graft.

The final feature of the cornea important to a consideration
of its transplantation immunobiology is the absence of blood
vessels and lymphatics in the normal corneal stroma. These
vessels are normally present only outside of the cornea at the
limbus, and even when neovascularization of the cornea does
occur, it tends to be restricted by the tight and well-ordered
meshwork of the corneal stroma.

THE SURVIVAL OF CORNEAL CELLS

The special privilege manifested by corneal transplants was
for many years ascribed to the replacement of donor cellular
elements by cells from the host, before immunologic sensitization
and/or attack could take place.[10] The frequent observation that

donor epithelium was sloughed from many grafts and rapidly
replaced by recipient cells, and the knowledge that the acellular
corneal stroma might yield a clear lamellar graft, seemed to lend
support to this conjecture. But beginning in 1960 with the
investigations of Basu,[11] numerous investigators were able to
demonstrate with sex chromatin,[12] tritiated thymidine,[13,14] or
karyologic markers[15,16] that all of the donor cellular elements
of the cornea might survive indefinitely in the recipient.
These studies are summarized elsewhere in this volume by Polack,
who himself has contributed importantly in this area.

ANTIGENICITY OF CORNEAL CELLS

The early impression that corneal grafts were insusceptible
to specific immunologic rejection led initially to suggestions
that corneal cells did not express transplantation antigens.[17,18]
This point was soon clarified by the demonstration that corneas
might be implanted into suitable vascular beds (e.g., subcutaneous
pockets), and in this site would induce rapid sensitization of
the host and rejection of the graft.[19,20] Even the corneal
epithelium, growing on a vascularized germinal site on the
rabbit but not itself invaded by recipient vessels, was able to
initiate the specific rejection process. It has been assumed
therefore, although not formally verified, that the several cell
types on the cornea display all of the histocompatibility
antigens included within the genome.

The occurrence on the surface of corneal cells of other
antigens which may contribute to various immunologic processes
by serving as recognition markers is less clear. It has been
reported that Ia antigen is expressed on a small number of cells
within the corneal epithelium,[21] but is lacking on keratocytes
and endothelial cells. Whether other significant antigens
encoded within the major histocompatibility complex are expressed
upon corneal cells is currently unknown: a complete investigation
of the distribution within the cornea of all of these antigenic
markers becomes increasingly more important for an understanding
of the transplantation immunobiology of the cornea.

CORNEAL GRAFT ADAPTATION

Only those changes which occur within a continuously viable
allograft to render it less immunogenic or more resistant to
rejection will be considered under this heading. The earliest

observation that suggested such a process was the finding of
Maumenee[7] that corneal allografts become less vulnerable to
rejection after a certain critical period of time. This concept
gained some currency both in corneal and in general tissue
transplantation from its strong sponsorship by Woodruff,[22]
based upon observations on graft survival within the anterior
chamber of the eye. More recent evidence, however, suggests
that the cause of these apparent changes is more likely due to
alterations in the host rather than changes in the graft.[23]
In sum, little convincing evidence has been presented in support
of the notion that a graft might undergo in situ adaptation,
and significant evidence has accumulated against this idea. Thus,
there is the frequent experimental and clinical observation that
a successful corneal graft may succumb to the specific rejection
process many months to years after surgery, and it has been
repeatedly observed (see below) that an experimental penetrating
graft in the rabbit may reside for many months on a recipient
corneal bed and then show full antigenicity and susceptibility
when retransplanted either to an ectopic location on the same
recipient or to a third-party recipient. It is probable,
therefore, that the "critical period" described in Maumenee's
study is to be attributed to the nonspecific healing-in of the
grafted cornea during the postoperative period, thus rendering
it less susceptible to physiologic embarrassment and the
resultant compromise of its immunologic privilege.

It may be appropriate here to comment upon the type of
graft "adaptation" which has been suggested to result from the
soaking of tissues in culture medium prior to their use as transplants (see Doughman, this volume). One explanation proposed
to explain the apparent benefits of this procedure has been that
the graft loses its passenger leukocytes during the soaking.[24]
However, the normal cornea, and especially the corneal graft
after passaging through a graft recipient, have no passenger
leukocytes, and yet retain full ability to stimulate the rejection
process. Alternatively, it has been suggested that soaking
somehow reduces the inherent antigenicity of the donor cells, but
again from the experiments described above it is unclear that
this takes place. Rather, soaking is generally found to reduce
the viability of the donor cellular elements, so that, at least

in the case of corneal grafts, it is not clear to what extent
donor cell viability is maintained.

THE IMMUNOLOGIC PRIVILEGE OF THE CORNEA

The discussion above has pointed out the reasons for
believing that the high success rate of corneal grafting is not
due to some innate privilege of the donor tissue itself. It
therefore becomes necessary to look to the recipient corneal
bed as the source of special immunologic privilege, in the
context of the general characteristics of immunologically
privileged sites as discussed in detail by Barker and
Billingham.[23]

Attention was called to the avascularity of the recipient
cornea as the principal basis for the immunologic protection of
an orthotopic corneal graft by Billingham and Boswell as early
as 1953.[19] Experience in both the clinic and the laboratory
has extensively confirmed this view, and indeed the degree of
vascularization of the recipient bed has long constituted one of
the major prognostic clinical criteria for graft success.[25-27]
Billingham and Boswell concluded that the absence of vessels in
the corneal graft provides an absolute barrier to the rejection
process, even in the sensitized host. But it is a familiar
observation that even a moderately vascularized corneal graft
may survive, so that it becomes necessary to define more
precisely the extent to which the privilege of corneal
transplants depends upon interference with the afferent limb of
sensitization as well as interruption of the efferent limb of
rejection.

The studies of Maumenee[7] showed early on that the survival
of corneal grafts may depend upon their inability to sensitize
the host. Maumenee found that technically successful penetrating
grafts would generally survive indefinitely in the experimental
rabbit, but that some 90% of these would fail after systemic
sensitization of the recipient with a skin graft from the
original donor. In follow-up studies to this, Khodadoust and
Silverstein[28] confirmed that while some 10% of avascular
penetrating grafts might be spontaneously rejected, the
remaining 90% failed to sensitize the host, since the rejection
of subsequent skin grafts from the same donor was not accelerated (Table I). In this study, systemic sensitization led to the

TABLE I. The effect of vascularization and of added host sensitization on the rejection of experimental lamellar and penetrating corneal allografts (adapted from Khodadoust and Silverstein[28]).

Graft	Vascular-ization	Added sensitiza-tion[a]	Percentage rejection	Mean rejection time of skin (days)
Lamellar	No	No	0	-
Lamellar	No	Yes	5	9.5
Lamellar	Yes	No	48	-
Lamellar	Yes	Yes	96	8.0
Penetrating	No	No	10	-
Penetrating	No	Yes	25	9.5
Penetrating	Yes	No	72	-
Penetrating	Yes	Yes	100	7.5

[a] Yes = orthotopic skin graft from same donor as cornea.

rejection of some 25% of well-established and clear grafts. However, when the experimental penetrating grafts were placed upon vascularized beds then 72% underwent specific rejection, the successful grafts induced partial sensitization of the host, and added systemic sensitization led to failure of all of the grafts. These data confirm the general impression that at least a portion of the immunologic privilege of the corneal graft may be accounted for by a defect in the afferent limb of sensitiza-tion, due to the normal absence of blood vessels in this tissue.

A degree of immunologic privilege also derives from an interference with the efferent limb of rejection provided by the avascularity of the cornea. We have already mentioned that rejection could be induced by systemic sensitization in only 25% of technically successful avascular penetrating corneal grafts in the rabbit. In the same study, it was found that systemic sensitization would promote the rejection of only 5% of successful lamellar grafts, a confirmation of an earlier report by Kornblueth and Nelken.[29] This finding not only confirms the better prognosis of lamellar grafts which lack the important and sensitive endothelial layer, but makes clear also the significant role of vascularization in mediating the rejection phase of the interaction of a host with its corneal graft.

But the vascularization of a recipient corneal bed is not an absolute guarantee that both sensitization and rejection of the corneal graft will occur. It is clear from the work of many investigators that the degree of vascularization constitutes one of the most important prognostic criteria for the success of corneal grafts, in that the more highly vascularized the bed, the more likely is the graft to be rejected, while the occasional graft may survive even upon a very highly vascularized recipient bed.

REJECTION OF INDIVIDUAL CELL LAYERS

In contrast to the rejection of orthotopic skin grafts, where rejection usually commences with the donor vascular endothelium and subsequent events are confusingly rapid and generally nonspecific concomitants of ischemia, experimental corneal grafts in the rabbit showed that corneal graft rejection might proceed very slowly, and involve the individual layers of the cornea separately and directly.[28,30,31] To study this more directly, techniques were devised permitting the orthotopic transplantation of pure corneal epithelium, corneal stroma, or substantially pure corneal endothelium in experimental rabbits. These experiments showed that not only were each of these cellular elements of the cornea independently capable of sensitizing the host and succumbing to specific rejection, but that the process could be followed over the course of a week to 10 days or more. Thus, the mechanism and cytology of the rejection process could be delineated more precisely than is possible with other solid tissue grafts. Moreover, it was found that the clinical course of rejection in each layer of the cornea might be so distinctive as to provide more useful criteria for the diagnosis of specific rejection of corneal grafts.

Pure corneal epithelium may be transplanted by transferring a deep lamellar graft without epithelium from one rabbit to another, permitting it to be reepithelialized by the recipient, and then cutting from the center of this graft a smaller and shallower lamellar button to be returned to the other eye of the original donor. If the epithelial graft is maintained avascular, it survives indefinitely. If, on the other hand, vessels are induced to grow to the graft margin, then sensitization and subsequent rejection may be induced. This takes the form of a

narrow line of epithelial rejection which starts in close
proximity to the nearest host vessels and slowly works its way
across the donor epithelial surface, destroying all donor cells
in its path (Fig. 2). The rejection process may take several
days to a week or more, and in the immediate area of donor
epithelial cell death, a mixture of lymphocytes and polymorpho-
nuclear leukocytes can be seen.[30,32]

Transplants of pure corneal stroma are readily performed by
the transplantation of a lamellar button of the cornea from
which the epithelium has been thoroughly scraped. Again, these
grafts survive indefinitely in the avascular recipient eye, but
rejection may be induced by encouraging vessels to invade the
cornea up to the graft margin. When this occurs, a broad band of
inflammatory cells (small and large lymphocytes with many poly-
morphonuclears) develops in that area of the graft adjacent to
the nearest host vessels (Fig. 3), and slowly sweeps across the
donor tissue leaving dead donor keratocytes in its wake.

The transplantation of pure corneal endothelium may be
effected using an approach similar to that adopted for epithelium.
In this instance, a very deep lamellar button with its own
epithelium is transplanted into a recipient bed from which all

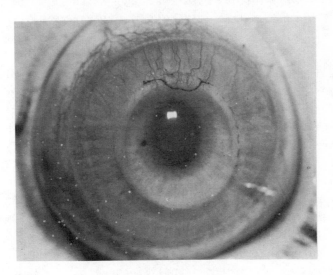

Figure 2. Rejection of corneal epithelium. The linear defect
is stained with topical methylene blue. (Reprinted with
permission from Khodadoust and Silverstein.[31])

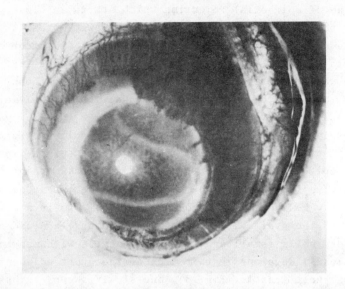

Figure 3. Rejection of corneal stroma. A dense band of
leukocytes moves from the vascularized edge of the graft toward
the avascular area. (Reprinted with permission from Khodadoust
and Silverstein.[30])

stroma has been carefully dissected down to the endothelial
basement membrane. After this graft has healed in, a smaller
penetrating graft is cut from its center and transferred to the
second eye of the original rabbit donor, so that only the
endothelial portion of the graft is foreign to the new recipient.
When, after healing in, this endothelial graft is caused to
become vascularized, then a line of endothelial destruction is
seen to start from the neighborhood of the nearest vessel, and
slowly spreads across the graft. In this instance, only
endothelial cells are destroyed, and stroma and epithelium is
left intact. But due to the physiologic importance of the
endothelium, the overlying corneal stroma becomes cloudy in step
with the endothelial destruction, and will remain cloudy until
endothelial healing takes place. Flat preparations of endothelium prepared during the course of the rejection process (Fig. 4)
show a narrow zone of predominantly mononuclear inflammatory
cells associated with endothelial cell destruction: behind this
zone, all endothelial cells are absent, while in front of this

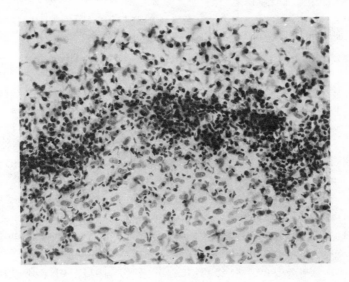

Figure 4. Rejection of corneal endothelium. Flat preparation, stained with hematoxylin. (Reprinted with permission from Khodadoust and Silverstein.[30])

zone normal endothelium can be seen. In no instance does the destruction of endothelium involve recipient endothelial cells beyond the margin of the graft.

THE MECHANISM OF REJECTION OF CORNEAL GRAFTS

The facts presented above make it evident that while the corneal graft does enjoy a certain degree of immunologic privilege due to its relative avascularity and also to certain structural features, yet it may be susceptible to immunologic rejection under certain circusmstances. Avascular recipient beds are not always available clinically, and even a clear cornea may at any time be compromised by a nonspecific insult leading to vascular- ization and a breakdown in both the afferent and efferent limbs of the rejection process. But the corneal transplant is unique in several respects, and it is these features that make it an ideal model for the transplantation biologist. First, the accessibility and transparency of the cornea make it easy to actually see many stages of the rejection process through the slit lamp microscope, a feature unavailable with other tissues. Secondly, the rejection process itself can be initiated at the whim of the investigator, by controlling vascularization of the

cornea and the degree of host sensitization. Thirdly, the
rejection process can be followed almost in slow motion over the
period of many days or even weeks, and in a structurally simple
tissue, permitting a more exact description of the cytology and
sequence of events than is possible with other solid tissue
grafts. Fourthly, the accessibility of the cornea makes it
possible to arrest the rejection process in mid-course in many
instances, by the application of topical corticosteroids.
Finally, the fact that the cornea does not require vascularization
for its function, and that those vessels that are found in a
rejecting graft are of recipient origin, means that the events
and destructive processes that accompany rejection of the cornea
are not the complicated byproducts of vascular damage and
ischemic necrosis such as is seen in rejecting grafts of skin,
kidney, and many other tissues. The simplicity of the corneal
rejection process is perhaps best illustrated by the graft-
versus-host reaction which occurs on the corneal endothelium
following inoculation into the anterior chamber of the rabbit eye
of appropriately sensitized lymphoid cells.[33,34] Some of these
cells find their way to the posterior (endothelial) surface of
the cornea, where they induce "pocks" of local endothelial
damage very reminiscent of the graft-versus-host reaction
described on the chorioallantoic membrane of the chick embryo.
Depending upon the dose of the donor cells administered, the
reaction may vary from only a few pocks to complete destruction
of the corneal endothelium. These pocks are easily visualized
as defects on the otherwise uniform mozaic of the endothelial
monolayer.

While it has been demonstrated[35] that lymphocytes, and
specifically T cells, can mediate graft rejection, the case made
for the participation of circulating antibodies has been less
satisfactory. One of the earliest suggestions[36] was that antibodies against blood group antigens present on corneal cells
might be involved in the rejection process. The suggestion has
also been made,[37] based upon in vitro studies, that cytotoxic
antibodies directed against tissue-specific antigens of the
cornea might play a role in the rejection process. However, an
examination of the data available on corneal graft rejection
in vivo, either clinical or experimental, indicates that as yet,

circulating antibodies have not been shown to be either necessary or sufficient to mediate corneal graft rejection.

ACKNOWLEDGEMENTS

This work was supported in part by United States Public Health Service Grant EY-00217 from the National Eye Institute, by an unrestricted gift from the Alcon Laboratories, Inc., and by an Independent Order of Odd Fellows Research Professorship.

REFERENCES

1. Medawar, P. B. 1944. Behaviour and fate of skin autografts and skin homografts in rabbits (report to War Wounds Committee of Medical Research Council). J. Anat. 78: 176.
2. Medawar, P. B. 1946. Immunity to homologous grafted skin: suppression of cell division in grafts transplanted to immunized animals. Brit. J. Exper. Path. 27: 9.
3. Billingham, R. E., L. Brent, and P. B. Medawar. 1954. Quantitative studies on tissue transplantation immunity: origin, strength and duration of actively and adoptively acquired immunity. Proc. Roy. Soc. Lond., B. 143: 58.
4. Woodruff, M. F. A. 1960. The Transplantation of Tissues and Organs. Charles C. Thomas, Springfield, Ill.
5. Leigh, A. G. 1966. Corneal Transplantation. Blackwell Scientific Publications, Oxford.
6. Paufique, L., G. F. Sourdille, and G. Offret. 1948. Les Greffes de la Cornée (Kératoplasties). Masson, Paris.
7. Maumenee, A. E. 1951. The influence of donor-recipient sensitization on corneal grafts. Am. J. Ophthalmol. 34: (Part II) 142.
8. Maumenee, A. E. 1955. The immune concept: its relation to corneal homotransplantation. Ann. N. Y. Acad. Sci. 59: 453.
9. Maumenee, A. E. 1962. Clinical aspects of the corneal homograft reaction. Invest. Ophthalmol. 1: 244.
10. Katzin, H. M. 1950. International Symposium on Corneal Surgery: Ultimate fate of the graft. Am. J. Ophthalmol. 33 2): 35.
11. Basu, P. K., I. Miller, and H. L. Ormsby. 1960. Sex chromatin as a biologic cell marker in the study of the fate of corneal transplants. Am. J. Ophthalmol. 49: 513.
12. Chi, H. H., C. C. Teng, and H. M. Katzin. 1965. The fate of endothelial cells in corneal homografts. Am. J. Ophthalmol. 59: 186.
13. Hanna, C., and E. S. Irwin. 1962. Fate of cells in the corneal graft. Arch. Ophthalmol. 68: 810.
14. Polack, F. M., G. K. Smelser, and J. Rose. 1964. Long-term survival of isotopically labeled stromal and endothelial cells in corneal homografts. Am. J. Ophthalmol. 57: 67.
15. Basu, P. K., P. Sarkar, and F. Carré. 1964. Use of the karyotype as biologic cell marker; in a study of immunologic reaction on the cellular elements of corneal heterografts. 58: 569.
16. Silverstein, A. M., A. M. Rossman, and A. S. de Leon. 1970. Survival of donor epithelium in experimental corneal xenografts. Am. J. Ophthalmol. 69: 448.

17. Bacsich, P., and G. M. Wyburn. 1947. The significance of the mucoprotein content on the survival of homografts of cartilage and cornea. Proc. Roy. Soc., Edinb., B. 62: 321.

18. Nelken, E., and D. Nelken. 1965. Serological studies in keratoplasty. Brit. J. Ophthalmol. 49: 159.

19. Billingham, R. E., and T. Boswell. 1953. Studies on the problem of corneal homografts. Proc. Roy. Soc., Lond. (Biol.) 141: 392.

20. Khodadoust, A. A., and A. M. Silverstein. 1966. Studies on the heterotopic transplantation of cornea to the skin. Survey Ophthalmol. 11: 435.

21. Klareskog, L., U. Forsum, U. M. Tjernlund, L. Rask, and P. A. Peterson. 1979. Expression of Ia antigen-like molecules on cells in the corneal epithelium. Invest. Ophthalmol. Visual Sci. 18: 310.

22. Woodruff, M. F. A. 1954. The "critical period" of homografts. Transplantation Bull. 1: 221.

23. Barker, C. F., and R. E. Billingham. 1973. Immunologically privileged sites and tissues. In Corneal Graft Failure, Ciba Foundation Symposium 15. Elsevier, Amsterdam.

24. Talmage, D. W., and H. Hemmingsen. 1975. Is the macrophage the stimulating cell? J. Allerg. Clin. Immunol. 55: 442.

25. Basu, P. K., and H. L. Ormsby. 1957. Studies of immunity with interlamellar corneal homografts in rabbits. Am. J. Ophthalmol. 44: 598.

26. Polack, F. M. 1962. Histopathologic and histochemical alterations in the early stages of corneal graft rejection. J. Exp. Med. 116: 709.

27. Khodadoust, A. A. 1973. The allograft rejection reaction: the leading cause of late failure of clinical corneal grafts. In Corneal Graft Failure, Ciba Foundation Symposium 15. Elsevier, Amsterdam.

28. Khodadoust, A. A., and A. M. Silverstein. 1972. Studies on the nature of the privilege enjoyed by corneal allografts. Invest. Ophthalmol. 11: 137.

29. Kornblueth, W., and E. Nelken. 1958. A study on donor-recipient sensitization in experimental homologous partial lamellar corneal grafts. Am. J. Ophthalmol. 45: 843.

30. Khodadoust, A. A., and A. M. Silverstein. 1969. Transplantation and rejection of individual cell layers of the cornea. Invest. Ophthalmol. 8: 180.

31. Khodadoust, A. A., and A. M. Silverstein. 1969. The survival and rejection of epithelium in experimental corneal grafts. Invest. Ophthalmol. 8: 169.

32. Kanai, A., and F. M. Polack. 1971. Ultramicroscopic alterations in corneal epithelium in corneal grafts. Am. J. Ophthalmol. 72: 119.

33. Khodadoust, A. A., and A. M. Silverstein. 1975. Local graft versus host reactions within the anterior chamber of the eye: the formation of corneal endothelial pocks. Invest. Ophthalmol. 14: 640.

34. Khodadoust, A. A., and A. M. Silverstein. 1976. Induction of corneal graft rejection by passive cell transfer. Invest. Ophthalmol. 15: 89.

35. Tagawa, Y., R. A. Prendergast, and A. M. Silverstein. In preparation.

36. Nelken, E., D. Nelken, I.C. Michaelson, and J. Gurevitch. 1961. Late clouding of experimental corneal grafts. Arch. Ophthalmol. 65: 584.
37. Manski, W., G. Ehrlich, and F. M. Polack. 1970. Studies on the cytotoxic immune reaction. I. The action of antibodies on normal and regenerating corneal tissues. J. Immunol. 105: 755.

The corneal graft reaction. An immunological, pathological and clinical perspective

Frank M.Polack, M.D.*

Department of Ophthalmology, University of Florida, Gainesville, Florida

ABSTRACT
        Graft rejection may be defined as cessation of function of
the transplant caused by immunological reactions. This phenomenon occurs in about 12-15% of all types of corneal transplants
in the human. This paper reviews the morphological and immunological alterations found in graft recipients. Histological
studies at the ultra structural level have been done in experimental animals, and they show the important role of lymphocytes
in the rejection process. The main characteristics of the clinical graft rejection are also reviewed with a discussion of the
role of cell mediated and humoral immune response.

INTRODUCTION

In 1960, when I first became interested in corneal trans-

plantation and its biological problems, little was known about

the various causes of graft failure, particularly the immune

graft rejection. In preparation for a research program planned

with George Smelser at that time, we reviewed the literature and

it was obvious that a confusion existed among clinicians as to

the causes of graft opacification. A few corneal surgeons re-

ported their techniques and the proper selection of cases for

corneal transplantation but no statistics were available as to

the number of successful grafts in various corneal diseases.

It was not infrequent to hear that corneal transplants opacified

two or three days after surgery due to graft reaction and the

term "graft sickness" was frequently used. This term derived

from the 1948 report on the cornea by Paufeque, Sourdille and

Offret[1], but even though Maumenee, in 1951[2], had identified the

time sequence and the early histological changes in the immune

graft reaction, the clinical picture of the disease and its his-

topathological features were by large unknown in the ophthalmic

literature. In 1945[3], the mechanisms of tissue rejection after skin transplantation had been discovered by Medawar, a discovery that was not accepted or recognized in all fields of medicine. It was believed at that time, that few cells in the graft survived after transplantation and that the death of transplanted cells were due to poor nutrition, replacement by host cells, and allergic reaction or death due to bacterial toxins.

In order to study the host-graft interaction it was important to determine if, in fact, transplanted cells survived for long periods of time after surgery. The demonstration of persistence of cell elements (cell antigens) in the donor tissue was important to understand the mechanisms of host versus graft reaction which could develop weeks, months or years after transplantation. Using isotopic labeling, we showed that the two most important layers in the cornea, the stromal and endothelial tissue, survived indefinitely after transplantation[4,5,6]. This was confirmed by other investigators also using isotopic labeling[7] or chromatin marking[8]. It was thus established that donor tissue could persist in the host cornea for long periods of time, as long as the host cornea was avascular. Further experiments showed that the lack of vascularization in the recipient cornea was the main reason for acceptance of a corneal graft rather than the lack of antigenicity of the donor tissue[9]. Host sensitization to a corneal graft was demonstrated in the experimental animal by the accelerated rejection of the first graft following a second graft; what is called a "second set phenomena" originally devised by Medawar and implemented in the eye by Maumenee in 1951[2]. Most of the experimental work on graft rejection has been done using this second set technique which allows the investigator to determine the time of rejection, thus facilitating the examination of rejecting grafts at different stages of the disease.

THE REJECTION OF CORNEAL HOMOGRAFTS

Graft rejection may be defined as cessation of function of the transplant caused by immunological reactions. In the cornea this is characterized by a progressive clouding of the corneal transplant in the absence of trauma or ocular disease[10]. A reasonable clinical diagnosis or corneal graft rejection can be made if a corneal transplant was clear prior to this episode of opacification. The incidence of graft reaction varies among other things with the pathological status or disease of the host cornea, ocular irritation by external physical agents or concomitant infectious disease. The incidence of graft rejection varies from 12 to 15% in good prognosis cases (mostly avascular corneas). It should be noted that in addition to the status of the host, the surgical technique, particularly problems with suturing or wound healing may increase the incidence of reactions[11,12,13].

ROLE OF HISTOCOMPATIBILITY ANTIGENS

The acceptance of a donor tissue depends on a large extent on the configuration and distribution of histocompatibility antigens in the cell membrane of the transplant. This is more important in highly vascularized tissues such as the kidney or liver. Histocompatibility or HLA antigens induce delayed hypersensitivity or the production of circulating antibodies. These antigens can be detected with a specific antisera. Even though an individual cannot have more than four antigenic determinants, each may have a series of different allo-antigens giving a total of over 127 HL-A variations. Transplantation antigens are located in the cell membrane and can be released without cell death as soon as the graft is implanted in the host tissue[14]. The lack of vascular channels in the cornea would not prevent these antigens from reaching the lymphoid tissue in a short period of time because antigens from the endothelial cells can be released into the aqueous humor which acts as a large vessel and the stromal antigens can diffuse through the interlamellar spaces to the limbal lymphatic capillaries. In regards to the donor tissue, it should be pointed out that alleles (other genes at the same locus) vary among ethnic groups. Such differences make proper selection of donor material more important when tissue originates from a donor of different ethnic origin. The importance of antigen A30 that runs in 30% of blacks, or the antigen A9 that occurs in 7% of whites and 31% of Japanese, is not known and deserves some investigation.

Histocompatibility studies on the cornea have been reported by several authors[16,17,18,19]. Results are conflicting as to the importance of perfect or partial antigen matching on the survival of corneal grafts. Blocking of these antigens with antibody has been suggested[20,21].

CELL MEDIATED IMMUNITY AND THE ROLE OF LYMPHOCYTES

It is assumed that once the antigens reach the lymphatic circulation or the lymph node, they are captured by macrophagues or by lymphocytes in the peripheral circulation. These cells are the small or the T lymphocytes that may originate clones of immunocompetent cells. They form the majority of circulating lymphocytes, the mediators of all hypersensitivities of the delayed type and are the effectors of graft rejection. The macrophages reaching the lymph node with donor antigens may also activate a group of lymphocytes which eventually will acquire the power to transfer sensitivity. There is histological evidence that lymphocytes can proliferate at the corneal limbus as immunocompetent cells and migrate through the host cornea into the transplanted tissue to cause the destruction of the cellular graft components[9]. The fact that graft reactions can be suppressed by the topical administration of steroids is a clear indication that these lymphocytes can be destroyed or neutralized in situ by the steriod therapy. The effect of topical steroids on immunocompetent lymphocytes engaged in graft rejection has been demonstrated experimentally[38]. It has also been shown, experimentally, that during the active graft rejection lymphocytes in different lymph nodes or lymphatic areas of the reticulo endothelial system appear to be hyperplastic and probably participate in the graft rejection phenomenon[34]. It is in these cases of systemic lymphocytic activation that systemic steroids seem to be indicated. It appears that most of the cell destruction in corneal grafts, as seen clinically or experimentally, occurs by direct contact of lymphocytes with the donor cells[39]. The exact mechanism of cell destruction is not known, but it is suspected that the lymphocyte will produce a rupture in the cell membrane of the donor cell. The ultramicroscopic pictures that will be shown below demonstrate only the final effect of lymphocyte action on the donor tissue but not the early injury on the donor cell.

HUMORAL HYPERSENSITIVITY AND GRAFT REJECTION

The role of circulating antibodies in corneal graft rejection is not well understood. This mechanism is effective by the so-called B lymphocytes which have abundant immunoglobulin (IgG) molecules. It is possible that in some instances, when graft rejection occurs rather diffusely and rapidly[22], the reaction may be mediated by immunoglobulins, as suggested by the studies of Manski et al.[23] They found a cytotoxic effect of anti-corneal antiserum only after the cells had been damaged or while they were regenerating, a situation that could parallel that of a recent graft. In our laboratory we found increased IgG concentrations in the aqueous humor of eyes of rabbits undergoing graft rejection,[13] suggesting that in some instances humoral antibodies may affect the endothelium of recent corneal transplants. The following studies give some information on the role of humoral antibodies in graft reaction.

Alberth et al.[24] using the passive-hemagglutination method of Boyden showed a regular sequence of appearance, rise and disappearance of antibody titer post operatively in 39 consecutive keratoconus patients. He was not able to correlate these events with the opacification and lasting transparency of the cornea.

Kapichnikov et al.[25] using immunothermistography and the microprecipitation test of Hoigne was able to demonstrate in laboratory animals that antibody titers became positive from the third day in 1/3 to 1/2 of their cases. There was a regular rise by the end of the first week that became maximal in three weeks. The titer remained high for about two months followed by a gradual decrease and disappearance within 4-6 months. They were able to further correlate the titer values with the status of the graft. In the clear and minimally cloudy grafts the antibody titer appeared later (7-10 days), amount was lower and had completely disappeared by six months. In the opaque grafts the titer appeared early, with reactions positive or very strongly positive.

Aviner and Henley[26] in their 1977 studies in patients with corneal allografts found that:

a) LMI test was positive in 75% of patients;

b) LMI developed during the third and fourth postoperative week and is usually not associated with rejection unless the cornea is vascularized;

c) LMI becomes negative in patients with successful transplant;

d) persistence of LMI after the first month in patients with clear graft is indicative of eventual graft reaction and failure.

The conclusion that can be inferred from their work is that systemic sensitization to corneal antigens occur early post operatively. Loss of LMI suggests that the graft becomes "isolated" after decrease of post operative tissue edema or inflammation, and the development of scar in the host/graft junction.

Our investigations have shown that with further modification the LIF assay may be a useful predictive index of graft rejection. Fifteen patients were tested preoperatively for LIF production in response to pooled corneal antigen. Of the four patients who later underwent rejection episodes, three had given positive LIF responses before surgery, while nine of the eleven patients without rejection had been negative for LIF production. It is possible that the one false negative and two false positive responses could be eliminated by the use of a better defined antigen.

MacDonald et al.[21] had previously used the ^{51}Cr release assay to demonstrate the role of complement independent cellular cytotoxicity factor in graft reaction. By using the same method they attempted to determine if antibodies released by bone marrow-derived immune lymphocytes in the presence of complement and unsensitized K (or null cells) can damage specific antibody coated donor cells. The ^{51}Cr assay was negative for these modalities and the workers felt that none of these factors play a major role in the destruction of donor corneal cells.

It is clear that data in the literature regarding the role of humoral antibodies is unclear and even contradictory. Most workers consider the role of humoral antibodies to be subsidiary in the rejection of allogenic and solid tumor grafts, but significant in the destruction of kidney grafts. To some extent this may be due to the sensitivity of the methods used to detect anti-corneal antibodies. These studies demonstrate the need for more work before definite conclusions can be drawn.

ROLE OF HOST VASCULARIZATION AND GRAFT REJECTION

I have mentioned above that the incidence of graft rejection ranges between 12% and 15% in avascular corneas or in eyes with good prognosis[10]. The prognosis of corneal transplantation depends upon the degree of pathology of the recipient cornea in which corneal vascularization plays a most important role[12-28]. It has been shown experimentally that host vascularization is essential for the experimental graft to be rejected[9]. We have also shown that the growth of vessels into the cornea usually brings along new lymphatic capillaries[13b, 29]. This combination

of blood vessels and lymphatic channels opens the door for antigens to be quickly released from the cornea and for immunocompetent cells to reach the corneal graft.

CRITERIA FOR DIAGNOSING AND ASSESSING AN ALLOGRAFT REJECTION
PROCESS[9, 10, 11, 12, 22]

There are several clinical parameters that may help to diagnose a graft rejection:

1. The process starts 3 weeks or more in a technically
   successful and clear graft.

2. The inflammatory process is limited primarily to
   the graft.

3. The process starts at the graft margin nearest to
   the most proximal blood vessels.

4. There is movement of inflammatory cells inward from
   its origin at the host-graft junction to involve
   the entire graft.

5. In a mild to moderate degree of severity, the typical
   pattern of an endothelial rejection band or line
   and/or a stromal rejection band may appear in
   25-30% of cases.

6. Frequently there is an increase in intraocular
   pressure.

It is difficult, clinically, to distinguish immunoallergic
graft reaction from "failure" due to operative and post operative
complications if the graft was not clear immediately after surgery. Rejections occurring within three (3) months are termed
"early rejections" and rejections occurring therafter are called
"late rejections"[10, 22, 28].

As mentioned before, the morbidity and characteristics of
the immune graft reaction vary with the condition of the recipient cornea (scarring, vascularization, active inflammation, previous grafts and other factors)[12], the immunologic status of the
host and a multitude of noncorneal conditions which may facilitate and accelerate graft reactions (dry eyes, lid closure defects, glaucoma, etc.)[22]. These conditions play vital roles,
especially in the early post operative period and partially explain the severity of early rejection. "Immunologic tolerance"
and/or "adaptation" account for the weaker reaction observed in
late rejections[10, 13, 22].

CLINICAL FEATURES OF GRAFT REJECTIONS[9-13, 22]

Early - Two patterns are recognized.

1) Diffuse graft edema with scattered K.P.'s; mild aqueous flare and edema of the posterior layer of the graft.

2) Graft edema or K.P.'s which begin near the scar adjacent to an area of vessel ingrowth, defective wound healing or irido-corneal adhesions. This form may show a typical rejection line.

The early graft rejection is usually severe and rapid, occurring generally in eyes with severe chemical burns, previous grafts, irido-corneal synechiae and active intraocular inflammation. Symptoms of graft reactions include: Ocular discomfort, photophobia and decreased or blurry vision. Slit lamp biomicroscopy may only show vascular engorgement (mostly around sutures), loss of epithelial luster, epithelial edema and epithelial defects. Graft thickness rapidly increases and K.P.'s soon appear; however, the amount of cells in the anterior chamber is not always proportionate to the degree or severity of the graft cloudiness. Deep vessels may start to invade the periphery of the graft stroma, which already show cellular infiltration[9, 12, 13, 22, 30, 31]. In about one-third (1/3) to one-half (1/2) of the cases a band of lymphocytic infiltration is present between the edge of the rejected and normal endothelium. This is called the "rejection line" and it is the only pathogromonic evidence of graft reaction.

Late graft reaction as a rule is less severe. The onset may go unnoticed by the patient and unsuspecting doctor. Symptoms can be so subtle that patients may go several days before seeking medical attention. Rejection usually begins in the scar with previous healing defect or iris synechiae[22]. The graft edema and infiltrate progress toward the center of the graft.

It is well recognized that the rejection process can involve any single layer of cornea or all layers at the same time[12]. The clinical picture of rejection in each layer is so distinctive as to be almost diagnostic. This is discussed by A. Silverstein elsewhere in this book.

Experimental studies of epithelial[30-32], stromal[9, 31, 33-35],

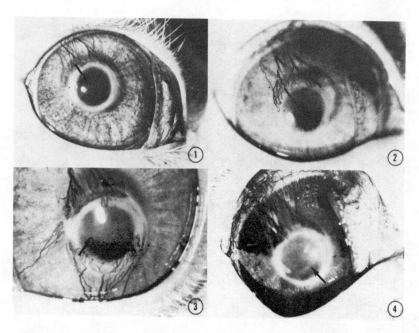

Fig. 1. A photograph of a clear rabbit homograft two weeks after operation.

Fig. 2. Crescent-shaped opacity of the graft adjacent to the vessels in the scar at the beginning of the rejection process.

Fig. 3. A photograph of a corneal homograft on the 2nd day of the rejection phenomenon. The graft shows peripheral edema and a horizontal hazy band midway between two sets of vessels.

Fig. 4. Graft rejection one week after the onset of opacification. Same eye as shown in Fig. 1.

or endothelial [9, 10, 27, 30-35] rejection have shown the participation of lymphocytes in the rejection process.

DISCUSSION

The immune graft reaction occupies a well defined and important place in corneal surgery even though it may be only one of the many causes of graft opacification. The biology of the corneal graft was studied in the early 60's and evidence was presented to show that the donor cells, particularly the corneal endothelium, could persist in the host for indefinite periods of time, as long as the immune reaction did not occur. These studies and the fact that clear corneal transplants could be ob-

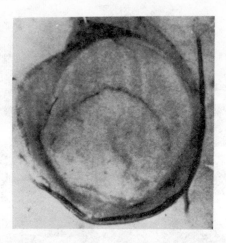

Fig. 5. Flat endothelial preparation showing partial destruction of the endothelium in the upper part of the graft. Round cells form a band which limits the end of the normal zone. Hematoxylin and eosin. (X15)

served in cases of endothelial dystrophy for many years after transplantation demonstrated that corneal transplants in fact behave as true chimeras. Our experimental studies of corneal heterografts as well as homografts have shown that the host can be sensitized to a small corneal transplant. Immunologic studies by several authors[24-27] and in our laboratory have shown that cell mediated immunity (CMI) as demonstrated by the lymphocyte migration inhibition test (LMIF), occurs in patients with corneal transplants, indicating that the recipients became sensitized to the corneal tissue. These authors found that in over 50% of the cases the LMI test was positive after transplantation, results that are similar to those obtained in our laboratory. The specificity of this test, however, is questionable since we and others had negative LMIF in cases of active graft rejection. Since the test is done with peripheral lymphocytes, it is possible that those lymphocytes surrounding the corneal graft (limbal) may be the effectors of rejection and few of those cells may be present in the sample harvested for the LMIF test. The mechanism by which donor cells are damaged during the rejection episode has not been demonstrated. The various factors that seem to influence the development of a graft rejection comprise: a) the structural condition of the recipient cornea and its avascularity; b) excessive donor tissue manipulation with loss of endothelial cells which may lead to graft edema facilitating the development of rejection if vascularization is stimulated by this persistent corneal edema; c) bad suturing techniques with monofixation of wound edges or incarceration of iris tissue opening the door for new vessels and the access of immunocompetent cells to the donor tissue.

In my experience the incidence of graft rejection can be reduced by the selection of fine suture material, small graft size (whenever possible), good donor tissue and perfect surgical technique. The proper use of steroids further reduces the incidence or severity of reactions.

REFERENCES

1. Polack, F. M., Smelser, G. K., and Rose, J. 1964. Long-term survival of isotopically labeled stromal and endothelial cells in corneal homografts. Amer. J. Ophthal. 57: 67.
2. Paufique, L., Sourdille, G. P., and Offyet, G. 1948. Les Gyeffes de la Cornee, Masson, Paris.
3. Maumenee, A. E. 1951. Influence of donor-recipient sensitization on corneal grafts. Amer. J. Ophthal. 34: 142.
4. Medawar, P. 1948. Immunity to homologous grafted skin III. The fate of skin homografts transplanted to the brain, to the subcutaneous tissue and anterior chamber of the eye. Brit. J. Exp. Path. 29: 58.
5. Polack, F. M. and Smelser, G. K. 1962. The persistence of isotopically labelled cells in corneal grafts. Proc. Soc. Exp. Biol. Med. 110: 60.
6. Polack, F. M. 1966. Four-year retention of ^{3}H thymidine by corneal endothelium. Arch. Ophthal. 75: 659.
7. Hanna C. and Irwin, E. S. 1962. Fate of cell in the corneal grafts. Arch. Ophthal. 68: 880.
8. Basu, P. K., Miller, I., and Ormesby, H. C. 1960. Studies on antigenicity of corneal heterografts. Amer. J. Ophthal. 49: 511.
9. Polack, F. M. 1962. Histopathological and histochemical alterations in the early stages of corneal graft rejection. J. Exp. Med. 116: 709.
10a. Inomata, H., Smelser, G. K., and Polack, F. M. 1970. The fine structural changes in the corneal endothelium during graft rejection. Invest. Ophthal. 9: 263.
10b. Polack, F. M. 1973. Clinical and pathological aspects of the corneal graft rejection. Trans. Amer. Acad. Ophth. 77: 418.
11. Maumenee, A. E. 1973. Clinical patterns of corneal graft failure. In Cornea Graft Failure - CIBA Symposium Excerpta Medica, Amsterdam, p. 5.

12. Khodadoust, A. A. 1973. The allograft rejection reaction: The leading cause of late 151 failure of clinical corneal graft. In Cornea Graft Failure - CIBA Foundation Symposium, p. 151.
13a. Polack, F. M. 1973. Corneal graft rejection: Clinico-pathological correlation. In Cornea Graft Failure - CIBA Foundation Symposium. 15: 128.
13b. Polack, F. M. 1973. Clinical patterns of corneal graft failure. In. Cornea Graft Failure - CIBA Symposium Discussion of Maumenee, A. E., p. 19.
14. Schwartz, B. D. and Mattheson, S. G. 1971. Regeneration of transplantation antigen on mouse cells. Transpl. Proc. 3: 180.
15. Bodmer, W. L. 1975. The HLA System presented at the John Hopkins Centenial Symposium on Genetics, Baltimore, MD.
16. Ehlers, N. and Ahrons, S. 1971. Corneal transplantation and histocompatibility. Acta Ophthal. 78: 61.
17. Stark, W. S., Opelz, G., Newsome, et al. 1973. Sensitization to human lymphocyte antigens by corneal transplantation. Invest. Ophthal. 12: 639.
18. Allansmith, M. R., Fine, M., and Pryne, R. 1974. Histocompatibility typing and corneal transplantation. Trans. Am. Acad. Ophthal. 78: 445.
19. Vannas. 1975. Histocompatibility in corneal grafting. Invest. Ophthal. 14: 883.
20. Chandler, J. W., Gebhardt, B. M., and Kaufman, H. E. 1973. Immunologic protection of rabbit corneal allografts: Preparation and in vitro testing of heterologus blocking antibody. Invest. Ophthal. 12: 646.
21. Binder, P. S., Gebhardt, B. M., Chandler, J. W., and Kaufman, H. E. 1973. Immunologic protection of rabbit corneal allografts with heterologous "blocking" antibody. Invest. Ophthal. 12: 646.
22. Polack, F. M. 1977. Corneal Transplantation. Grune and Stratton, a subsidiary of Harcourt, Brace, Javonovish, Publishers New York, San Francisco, London.
23. Manski, W., Ehrlich, G., and Polack, F. M. 1970. Studies on the cytotoxic immune reaction: I. The action of antibodies on normal and regenerating corneal tissue. J. Immunol. 105: 755.
24. Alberth, B. et al. 1974. Anticorneal antibody examination in Human Keratoplasty. Albrecht v. Graefes Arch. Clin. Exp. Ophthal. 190: 340.
25. Kapichnikov, M. M. et al. 1975. The use of immunothermistography as a method of detecting humoral antibodies following allografting of skin and cornea in rabbits. Bull. Enp. Biol. Med. 80. 8: 948.
26. Aviner, Z. and Henley, W. L. 1977. Leucocyte Migration Inhibition Test in ocular surgery. Ophthalmic Surgery. 8: 51.
27. MacDonald, A., Ohashi, K., and Basu, P. K. 1978. Are serum antibody complement or K-cell dependent cellular cytotoxicity involved in corneal graft rejection? Can. J. Ophthal. 13: 182.
28. Fine, M. and Stein, M. 1973. The role of corneal vascularization in human corneal graft reactions 193. In Cornea Graft Failure - CIBA Foundation Symposium.
29. Inomata, H., Smelser, G. K., and Polack, F. M. 1970. Fine structure of regenerating endothelium and Descemet's membrane in normal and rejecting corneal grafts. Amer. J. Ophthal. 70: 48.
30. Silverstein, A. M. and Khodadoust, A. A. 1973. Transplantation immunobiology of the cornea 105. In Cornea Graft Failure - CIBA Foundation Symposium.

31. Kanai, A. and Polack, F. M. 1971. Ultramicroscopic changes in the corneal graft stroma during early rejection. Invest. Ophthal. 10: 415.

32. Polack, F. M. 1972. Scanning electron microscopy of the corneal rejection: I. Epithelial rejection. II. Endothelial rejection. III. The formation of retrocorneal membranes. Invest. Ophthal. 11: 1.

33. Polack, F. M. 1966. Modification of the immune graft response by azathioprine. Surv. Ophthal. 11: 545.

34. Polack, F. M. 1966. The pathological anatomy of corneal graft rejection. Surv. Ophthal. 11: 391. (Also, Acta XX Concilium Ophthal., Germany, 1966, p. 885.)

35. Khodadoust, A. A. and Silverstein, A. M. 1969. The survival and rejection of epithelium in experimental corneal transplants. Invest. Ophthal. 8: 180.

36. Khodadoust, A. A. and Silverstein, A. M. 1969. Invest. Ophthal. 8: 169.

37. Polack, F. M. and Kanai, A. 1972. Electron microscopic studies of the graft endothelium in corneal graft reactions. Amer. J. Ophthal. 73: 711.

38. Maumenee, A. E. 1973. The role of steroids in the prevention of corneal graft failure. In Cornea Graft Failure - CIBA Foundation Symposium.

39. Polack, F. M. 1973. Lymphocyte destruction during corneal homograft reaction. A scanning electron microscopic study. Arch. Ophthal. 89: 413.

*Dr Polack was unable to attend the workshop because of a medical emergency. This is his prepared presentation.

Keratoplasty: the role of histocompatibility (HLA) antigens

Walter J.Stark, M.D., Hugh R.Taylor, M.D., A.Edward Maumenee, M.D. and Wilma B.Bias, Ph.D.

The Wilmer Ophthalmological Institute, The Johns Hopkins Medical Institutions, Baltimore, Maryland 21205

ABSTRACT

Allograft rejection is one of the leading causes of corneal graft failure in man when the cornea is heavily vascularized. This paper reports the feasibility and possible benefits of using histocompatibility (HLA) antigen cross-match testing for corneal donor selection. Such cross-match testing does not require the matching of individual HLA antigens of donor and recipient. A double-masked clinical trial designed to determine the value of this procedure for keratoplasty is discussed.

INTRODUCTION

The incidence of corneal allograft rejection varies con-siderably, depending in part on the degree of vascularization of the recipient corneal bed. In avascular recipient corneas, rejection occurs in 2.3% to 35% of cases[1-3]. However, when the recipient cornea is densely vascularized, rejection develops in up to 65% of cases[1,4]. In such cases in which vasculariza-tion is dense, about 50% of grafts undergoing a rejection-reaction result in graft failure[1,2]. Therefore, with recent improvements in surgical techniques it appears that allograft rejection is now the greatest cause of delayed corneal graft failure in man[1].

In cases of allograft rejection after keratoplasty, the precise role of donor-recipient histocompatibility (HLA) antigens is not fully known. Some authors have found a significant correlation between the number of matching donor and recipient HLA antigens and the graft results in high-risk cases of vascularized corneas[4,5], but other studies have not shown a similar correlation[6].

The HLA antigen system is the major transplantation antigen system in man, as demonstrated by analysis of familial renal transplantation results[7,8]. Because of the complexity of the HLA antigen system, the probability for complete matching of donor and recipient antigens for unrelated (non-familial) cadaver transplants is low. In renal transplantation, the presence of preimmunization of the recipient to HLA antigens of the donor increases the risk of rejection[9-13]. However, in cases of keratoplasty the effect of recipient preimmunization has not been fully evaluated.

It is known that patients can become immunized and develop lymphocytotoxic antibodies -- by exposure to foreign HLA antigens from previous transplants (including corneal transplants, as we have reported[14]) or blood transfusions[10], or pregnancy[15]. Preimmunization of the recipient to antigens of the donor may be detected by preoperative cross-match testing between the recipient's serum and the donor's lympho-cytes[13,16]. A negative cross-match test indicates that the recipient has no circulating lymphocytotoxic antibodies specific for the antigens of the donor, whereas a positive cross-match test indicates that the recipient has previously been sensitized and developed antibodies to one or more antigens of the donor. A positive donor-recipient cross-match before renal transplantation almost always results in hyper-acute allograft rejection[13,16].

The purpose of this paper is to present further data on the outcome of penetrating keratoplasty in 86 potentially-preimmunized recipients with severe preoperative corneal vascularization[17], and also to report the results of HLA cross-match testing and specific-antigen matching.

The donor corneas that were used for the keratoplasty cases were selected on the basis of obtaining a negative donor-recipient cross-match test before surgery. No attempt was made in these cases to match donor and recipient HLA antigens specifically (for each individual antigen).

MATERIALS AND METHODS

Eighty-six penetrating keratoplasties were performed on this series of study patients between November 1973 and November 1978. Patients selected for this study had significant vascularization of the corneal stroma in at least three quadrants, extending into the visual axis. Of the 86 patients studied, 64 (74%) had previously had at least one corneal transplant failure in that same eye. These 64 patients had an average of 1.9 previous graft failures, with a range of from 1 to 6 previous graft failures in that eye. The remaining 22 patients had previously been exposed to foreign HLA antigens by keratoplasty in the other eye or by blood transfusion or pregnancy. Of the 86 patients, 51 were female and 35 were male. The age of recipients ranged from 13 years to 80 years (mean, 60 years).

Preoperatively, sera from all waiting keratoplasty patients were cross-matched individually against lymphocytes of all the potential corneal donors. A specific donor cornea for an individual recipient was selected on the basis of a

negative cross-match reaction with the donor's lymphocytes.
If a positive cross-match was obtained, the cornea was not used
for that recipient, because a positive cross-match indicates
that the recipient has antibodies that are specific for one or
more antigens of that donor. In addition, HLA typing of both
donor and recipient was obtained but no attempt was made to
match donor and recipient for each individual antigen specifically.

The diagnosis of immune graft rejection was made only if
the graft remained clear for at least 2 weeks after surgery
and then developed edema or clouding associated with keratic
precipitates on the graft endothelium, or a rejection line.
Non-immune causes of graft failure included grafts that clouded
within 2 weeks of surgery, or graft clouding associated with
infection, trauma, glaucoma, or persistent epithelial defects
with exposure keratitis.

RESULTS AND COMMENTS

1. Negative Donor-Recipient Cross-Match Pairs:

Results: Postoperatively 67 of the 86 corneal grafts
(78%) are clear, with an average follow-up of 15.6 months
(range 6 to 45 months). Fifteen percent of the grafts (13 of
86) have failed from immune allograft rejection, and 7% have
failed from causes other than rejection (Table 1). Twelve
of the thirteen graft failures from rejection occurred
within 6 months of surgery, with the average time for
occurrence of rejection being 3.6 months. Twenty-two of the
86 patients (26%) had evidence of an immune event, either
rejection or a reversible allograft reaction. Nine of the 22
immune events could be reversed with corticosteroids,

TABLE 1 Outcome of keratoplasty in potentially preimmunized recipients with dense corneal vascularization: Negative donor-recipient cross-match

Total	Allograft rejection	Non-immune graft failure	Total clear	Mean follow-up (range-months)
86	13 (15%)	6 (7%)	67 (78%)	15.6 (6-45)

TABLE 2 Immune reactions in potentially preimmunized recipients with dense corneal vascularization

Total No. of grafts	Total No. of immune events (rejection or reaction)	Allograft reaction (graft clear)	Percentage reversed
86	22 (26%)	9	41%

and 13 of the cases progressed to graft clouding (Table 2).

Comment: In these 86 keratoplasty cases with dense corneal vascularization, our incidence of graft rejection, which was 15%, is less than that reported in similar high-risk cases. Khodadoust[1] has reported graft failure from rejection in 65% of cases with dense corneal vascularization, and Batchelor and co-workers[4] reported 60% of such cases with graft failure from rejection. Although there may have been differences between their series and ours in factors such as the quality of donor material, or patient follow-up availability, these factors are unlikely to account for all of the large difference in incidence of rejection failures between those series and ours. A major cause of the lower incidence of rejection in our series is probably our use of negatively

cross-matched donor material. These findings for keratoplasty
are in agreement with the results in other tissue and organ
transplantation systems[13,16].

2. Retrospective Donor-Recipient HLA Antigen Matching:

Results: The donor and recipient HLA typing results were
known for the 86 cases that received negative cross-matched
grafts. There were 17 additional cases for whom the donor and
recipient HLA types were known. These additional 17 cases
also had dense corneal vascularization, but the cross-match
test had not been performed. The donor-recipient HLA antigen
matching was analyzed retrospectively for these 103 cases.

The occurrence of graft rejection was compared with the
number of matching donor and recipient antigens as shown in
Table 3. When the donor and recipient shared no matching
antigens, rejection failures occurred in 14% of the cases (7
of 51). When one matching antigen was shared, rejection
developed in 18% of cases (6 of 34). In 11 cases in which the
donor and recipient shared two matching antigens, we had no
graft failures from rejection. However, rejection accounted
for failure in 2 of 5 cases (40%) in which three matching
antigens were shared. We have only one case in which the donor

TABLE 3   Donor-Recipient HLA Antigen Matches and Graft Outcome

Number of HLA Antigens Matched	Number of Patients	Allograft Rejection	Nonimmune Graft Failure	Clear Graft
0	51	7(14%)	5(10%	39(76%)
1	35	6(17%)	1(3%)	28(80%)
2	11	0	0	11(100%)
3	5	2(40%)	0	3(60%)
4	1	0	0	1(100%)
Total	103	15(15%)	6(6%)	82(80%)

and recipient shared four matching antigens, and this graft is clear.

Thus, the incidence of graft failure from rejection does not correlate clearly and consistently with the number of matching HLA antigens shared between the donor and recipient. Also, the incidence of immune events and the reversibility of allograft reaction did not appear to correlate with the number of antigens shared (Table 4).

Comment: Batchelor and co-workers[4] have the largest series published to date regarding donor-recipient HLA antigen matching and the graft outcome. In 73 keratoplasty recipients with dense corneal vascularization, they showed a reduction in graft failure from rejection as the donor and recipients shared increasingly-more matched antigens. Our work does not confirm this in similar high-risk cases (Figure 1). However, the majority of our cases received corneas from negatively cross-matched donors. Batchelor did not report having used cross-match testing for donor selection, although the probability of negative cross-matches will obviously be higher with donor-recipient pairs that are well-matched for specific antigens.

TABLE 4   Donor-Recipient HLA Antigen Match and Graft Outcome

Number of HLA Antigens Matched	Number of patients	Total Number of Immune Events (Reaction or Rejection)	Allograft Reaction (Graft Clear)	Percent Reversed
0	51	14(27%)	7	50
1	35	9(26%)	3	33
2	11	1(9%)	1	100
3	5	2(40%)	0	0
4	1	0	0	--
Total	103	26(25%)	11	42

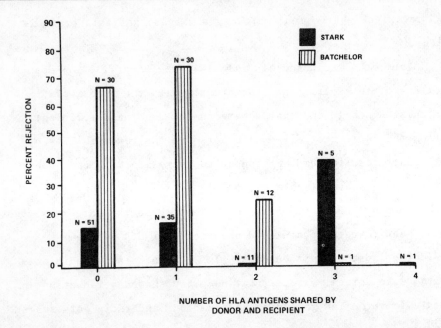

Fig. 1 (Stark and associates). The incidence of rejection
after keratoplasty in recipients who have shared zero, one,
two, three or four HLA antigens with their donor. Comparison
between this study and that of Batchelor and co-workers[4].
(Reprinted with permission, Stark, W.J., Taylor, H.R., and
Bias, W.B.: Histocompatibility (HLA) antigens and keratoplasty.
AJO 86:595-604, 1978).

DISCUSSION AND CONCLUSIONS

It is not known whether humoral immunity plays a role in

corneal graft rejection. Previous work suggests that corneal

graft rejection is mediated by cellular immune responses[18].

However, in either case, the HLA serologic reactions can be

used as indicators of recipient preimmunization, because the

major gene loci controlling cell-mediated responses also map

within the HLA complex. Thus far, about 10 loci, all control-

ling some aspect of immune function, have been assigned to the

HLA region of chromosome 6 in man[19]. The D locus (or subregion) controls mixed lymphocyte responsiveness, and is an in-vitro indicator of cellular immune responsiveness. The entire HLA complex occupies a very small segment of the chromosomal length, allowing one to characterize a given haplotype (the gene complex on one chromosome of the pair) by the serologic specificities it contains.

Our results show a lower incidence of corneal graft failure from rejection when cross-match testing was used for donor selection than did other series involving similar high-risk cases with dense corneal vascularization[1,4]. We believe this difference is due mainly to our use of preoperative donor-recipient cross-match testing as a means for donor selection. By so doing, we are able to avoid giving a donor cornea to a recipient who happens to be presensitized to one or more of that cornea's antigens[20].

Although we found no consistent correlation between the number of matching HLA antigens shared between the donor and recipient regarding the graft outcome, the role of specific antigen matching may still deserve further evaluation. However, if further attempts at donor-recipient HLA antigen matching are to be made they should be combined with preoperative cross-match testing, because even if all but one of the known donor-recipient antigens are favorably matched, the recipient still might happen to be preimmunized to the one unmatched donor antigen, or perhaps to donor HLA antigens that are not yet known. Although perfect donor-recipient HLA matching for corneal transplantation may be beneficial, it is not at this time practical because of the complexity of the HLA system[21]. Our study, however, demonstrates that the use of nonspecific cross-matching to avoid donors with transplantation antigens to which the recipient is immunized is feasible and seems beneficial.

This study shows the feasibility of using negative cross-match testing for donor selection in keratoplasty; but since we did not have positive donor-recipient cross-match controls in this study, we consider this to be a preliminary report. A double-masked clinical trial is currently underway to determine the value of donor selection based on histocompatibility (HLA) antigen cross-match testing for keratoplasty in high-risk cases. In the controlled study, keratoplasty recipients with dense corneal vascularization and detectable lymphocytotoxic antibodies will be randomized into two groups. One group will receive corneas from a positively cross-matched donor (lymphocytotoxic antibodies of recipient are specific for one or more HLA antigens of the donor), and the other group will receive corneas from a negatively cross-matched donor (antibodies of recipient are not specific for any HLA antigens of the donor). Graft outcome will be carefully followed to determine the long-term effects of recipient pre-immunization. If this controlled study demonstrates that cross-match testing for donor selection has a favorable influence on the outcome of keratoplasty in recipients with densely-vascularized corneas, then cross-match testing should be routinely performed in such cases. Since these procedures are expensive and time-consuming, however, cross-match testing and antibody screening should not be adopted as routine until they have been scientifically proven to be of value.

ACKNOWLEDGEMENTS

This work was supported in part by the National Eye Institute, Grant EY01302 (Dr. Stark).

REFERENCES

1. Khodadoust, A. A. 1973. The allograft rejection reaction: the leading cause of late failure of clinical corneal grafts. In: Corneal Graft Failure, Ciba Foundation Symposium, Elsevier, Amsterdam, p. 151.
2. Stark, W. J., D. Paton, A. E. Maumenee, P. E. Michelson. 1972. The results of 102 penetrating keratoplasties using 10-0 monofilament nylon suture. Ophth. Surg. 3: 11.
3. Chandler, J. W., H. E. Kaufman. 1974. Graft reactions after keratoplasty for keratoconus. Am. J. Ophthalmol. 77: 543.
4. Batchelor, J. R., T. A. Casey, D. C. Gibbs, D. F. Lloyd, A. Werb, S. S. Prasad, and A. James. 1976. HLA matching and corneal grafting. Lancet 1: 551.
5. Vannas, S., K. Karjalainen, P. Ruusuvaara, and A. Tiilikainen. 1976. HLA-compatible donor cornea for prevention of allograft reaction. Graefe Arch. Ophthal. 198: 217.
6. Allansmith, M. R., M. Fine, R. Payne. 1974. Histocompatibility typing and corneal transplantation. Tr. Am. Acad. Ophthalmol. Otolaryngol. 78: 445.
7. Opelz, G., M. R. Mickey, P. I. Terasaki. 1977. Calculations on long-term graft and patient survival in human kidney transplantation. Transpl. Proc. 9: 27.
8. Mickey, R. M., M. Kreisler, E. D. Albert, N. Tanaka, and P. I. Terasaki. 1971. Analysis of HL-A incompatibility in human renal transplants. Tissue Antigens 2: 57.
9. Terasaki, P. I., M. Kreisler, R. M. Mickey. 1971. Presensitization and kidney transplant failures. Postgrad. Med. J. 47: 89.
10. Opelz, G., P. I. Terasaki. 1971. Histocompatibility matching utilizing responsiveness as a new dimension. Transpl. Proc. 4: 433.
11. Opelz, G., D. P. S. Sengar, R. M. Mickey, and P. I. Terasaki. 1973. Effect of blood transfusions on subsequent kidney transplants. Transpl. Proc. 5: 253.
12. Opelz, G., R. M. Mickey, and P. I. Terasaki. 1972. Identification of unresponsive kidney-transplant recipients. Lancet 1: 868.
13. Terasaki, P. I., D. L. Thrasher, T. H. Hauber. 1968. Serotyping for homotransplantation. XIII. Immediate kidney transplant rejection and associated preformed antibodies. In: Advance in Transplantation. Edited by J. Dausset, J. Hamburger, G. Mathe. Baltimore, Williams and Wilkins, p. 225.
14. Stark, W. J., G. Opelz, D. Newsome, R. Brown, R. Yankee, and P. I. Terasaki. 1973. Sensitization to human lymphocyte antigens by corneal transplantation. Invest. Ophthalmol. 12: 639.
15. Dausset, J. 1954. Leuco-agglutinins. IV. Leuco-agglutinins and blood transfusion. Vox Sang. 4: 190.

16. Kissmeyer-Nielsen, F., S. Olsen, V. Posborg-Petersen, and O. Fjeldborg. 1966. Hyperacute rejection of kidney allografts associated with pre-existing humoral antibodies against donor cells. Lancet 2: 662.
17. Stark, W. J., H. R. Taylor, W. B. Bias, and A. E. Maumenee. 1978. Histocompatibility (HLA) antigens and keratoplasty. Am. J. Ophthalmol. 86: 595.
18. Polack, F. M., and C. E. Gonzales. 1968. The response of the lymphoid tissue to corneal heterografts. Arch. Ophthalmol. 80: 321.
19. Bias, W. B., and S. H. Hsu. 1977. HLA, the major histo-compatibility system in man: An overview. Acta Anthropogen-etica 1: 15.
20. Newsome, D. A., M. Takasugi, K. R Kenyon, W. J. Stark, and G. Opelz. 1974. Human corneal cells in vitro: morphology and histocompatibility (HL-A) antigens of pure cell populations. Invest. Ophthalmol. 13: 23.
21. World Health Organization Committee. 1978. Nomenclature for factors of the HLA system 1977. Tissue Antigens 11: 81.

Transplantation of homologous corneal endothelium derived from tissue culture

James P.McCulley, M.D., David M.Maurice, Ph.D. and Barry D.Schwartz, Ph.D.

Division of Ophthalmology, Stanford University Medical School, Stanford, California 94305

ABSTRACT

The relative inadequacy of supply of donor corneas and the large number of patients with corneal edema alone accounting for decreased visual acuity, who would require only repopulation of the endothelial surface, led us to evaluate the transplantation of the endothelial layer alone using cells derived from tissue culture (TC) as a donor source. Other potential advantages to such a technique include decreased antigenic challenge and transplantation of mitotically active cells.

Seeding of stromal tissue with cells from TC has previously been shown to be an effective donor source. To more closely approach the ideal of transplanting the endothelium alone to autologous stroma, a membrane was developed which would support the growth of TC corneal endothelial cells and survive surgical manipulation. This membrane, with attached cells, has been transplanted to autologous stroma with a high degree of success.

INTRODUCTION

A major advance in corneal transplantation is being approached with the development of techniques for the transplantation of tissue cultured corneal endothelium. Both homologous[1-4] and heterologous[5,6] corneal endothelium has been maintained in tissue culture and subsequently successfully transplanted in animals. The potential clinical application of this in man is in patients who have poorly functional endothelium resulting in corneal edema before corneal scarring has resulted. In such patients the repopulation of the endothelial lining with healthy functional cells would result in deturgescence of the cornea. If no scarring had previously occurred, the cornea could recover normal clarity. The potential advantages to this technique over standard penetrating keratoplasty include ready availability of donor material, transplantation of a quantitatively and qualitatively lesser antigenic load, and transplantation of mitotically active cells in contrast to the normally inactive corneal endothelium of cadaver donor corneas.

There are two major obstacles to the realization of this ideal. One is the growth of endothelium in tissue culture; however, techniques have been developed[7,8] and modified[2,5,9] so that corneal endothelial cells from several animals have been successfully grown in tissue culture. Human cells have been grown with more difficulty.[10] However, there is much still to be done in this area.

The second major problem is the actual transplantation of the endothelial layer alone. Techniques have been developed such that it has been possible to transplant homologous rabbit endothelium into rabbits[1-4] or heterologous bovine endothelium into rabbits or other animals.[5,6] The techniques have included seeding of endothelial cells from tissue culture onto stroma denuded of its native endothelium. This stroma, seeded with cells from tissue culture has successfully served as a donor source in standard penetrating keratoplasty operations.[1,2,3,5,6] The limiting factor, preventing these techniques from being applied safely in procedures using autologous stroma, has been the time required for the tissue cultured cells to attach to the stromal substrate. The longer the seeding time the more likely the development of significant complications such as infection, intraocular hemorrhage, choroidal detachment, hypotony, or cataract formation.

A thin membrane on which endothelial cells could be grown was therefore developed.[3,11] Preliminary results using this membrane as substrate and carrier for tissue cultured endothelium in otherwise autologous penetrating keratoplasties have been reported.[4] The expanded series using this membrane seeded with tissue cultured endothelial cells as a donor source in otherwise autologous penetrating keratoplasties will be reported herein.

MATERIALS AND METHODS

Tissue culture: Rabbit corneal endothelial cells were established and maintained by methods previously reported.[2,9] Cells were labelled with tritiated thymidine and seeded onto a crosslinked gelatin membrane.

Membrane formation: A membrane which could serve as substrate for tissue cultured corneal endothelial growth was prepared by crosslinking gelatin with glutaraldehyde which resulted in a 1-5 μm thick, transparent, permeable, wrinkle-free membrane which will support the growth of tissue cultured corneal endothelial cells and is sufficiently strong to withstand surgical manipulation. The details of the procedure for forming this membrane have been previously reported in detail.[11] Currently a membrane approximately 1 μm thick is being used in all procedures. The membranes are currently made within a 13 mm cut-out in millipore filter so that it is possible to mount them in a modified Sykes-Moore chamber.

Attachment of membrane to autologous stroma: A saturated solution of gelatin, platelets-fibrinogen-thrombin, polysaccharides, amino acids, fibronectin, and cyanoacrylate, have been evaluated as adhesives for attachment of the membrane to autologous stroma. Of the substances tested to date, only cyanoacrylate provides a sufficiently firm adhesion to allow successful transplantation of the gelatin membrane. It has been possible to decrease the toxicity of the cyanoacrylate by using butylcyanoacrylate rather than methyl- or ethyl- and by diluting the butylcyanoacrylate with two parts of methylene chloride to one part butylcyanoacrylate.

The autologous stromal button at the time of surgery has native endothelium alone or in combination with Descemet's membrane removed. It is then placed posterior suface down on a membrane mounted in a Sykes-Moore chamber. Membrane and cornea are glued to one another by applying a minute amount of diluted butylcyanoacrylate in such a way that a peripheral rim of adhesion is formed between corneal stroma and membrane (Fig. 1).

Surgical procedure: The pupils of 10-12 lb. New Zealand albino female rabbits were dilated and the animals heparinized as previously described.[2] They were then placed under general anesthesia using a combination of chlorpromazine and ketamine intramuscularly. Tubing was placed in the anterior chamber to provide continuous flow of tissue culture medium

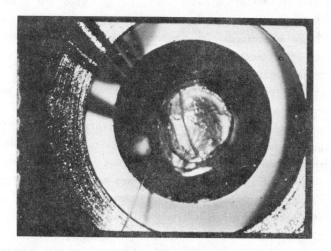

Figure 1 - A thin membrane crosslinked with glutaraldehyde and detoxified is shown mounted within a 13 mm cut-out in millipore filter, both of which are mounted in a modified Sykes-Moore chamber. An autologous stromal button is shown placed posterior surface down on this membrane. Small segments of cornea are sequentially elevated such that diluted butylcyanoacrylate adhesive can be applied creating an almost continuous thin rim of adhesion between peripheral cornea and membrane.

containing heparin throughout the surgical procedure. A 6.5 mm stromal button was obtained by trephination. Corneal endothelium alone or in combination with Descemet's was mechanically removed. The denuded autologous stromal button was glued to a membrane mounted in a Sykes-Moore chamber as described above. The membranes were either free of cells or had previously been seeded with homologous corneal endothelium as described above. The chamber was partially dismounted so that the autologous stromal button with attached membrane could be trephined free of excess membrane. The corneal button with attached membrane was replaced in the corneal bed and sutured in place with a continuous 10-0 nylon suture. Postoperatively, the animals received topical mydriatic cycloplegics, antibiotics, and subconjunctival steroids for 2-3 weeks.

The animals were examined at the slit lamp biomicroscope at which time corneal thickness was determined by pachometry on the operated as well as contralateral normal cornea 2-3 times per week. Periodically the lids were occluded for several hours using either lid sutures or a head wrap so that corneal thinning secondary to evaporation could be ruled out as the principal force thinning the cornea.

<u>Scintillation Counts</u>: At variable periods after surgery ranging up to 7 months, animals were sacrificed and membranes dissected free of stroma. These membranes with attached cells were then prepared for scintillation counting so that the origin of the cells on the posterior surface of the membrane could be determined. The portions of membranes with attached cells which remained after trephination of membrane which was glued to autologous stroma for transplantation, served as a source for baseline counts.

<u>Controls</u>: A positive control consisting of a complete autologous corneal transplant was done. The procedure followed exactly that which was followed when membrane was attached with the exception that the cornea was removed, placed in a sterile dish containing tissue culture medium for a 10-minute period, then replaced in the eye without removal of endothelium or attachment of membrane. A negative control was performed consisting of the removal of native endothelium with the attachment of a membrane which had not been seeded with endothelial cells.

RESULTS

<u>Attachment of membrane to autologous stroma</u>: The only adhesive which was adequate for attachment of membrane to cornea was diluted or undiluted cyanoacrylate. The one which proved to be the least toxic and yet still adequate was butylcyanoacrylate diluted with 2 parts methylene chloride. The method of application which proved to be the most successful resulted in

the formation of a peripheral rim of adhesion between membrane and stroma. If only native endothelium was removed leaving Descemet's membrane intact, a central fluid space would persist between membrane and stroma for approximately 10-12 days, after which it would rapidly disappear. If, in addition to removal of native endothelium, Descemet's membrane was removed, no such fluid space occurred, i.e., membrane was attached to overlying stroma at the time of surgery and remained attached throughout the period of observation.

The time lapse between removal of the corneal button to replacement with attached membrane averaged 10 minutes. During this time native endothelium alone, or in combination with Descemet's membrane, was removed. Membrane and cornea were glued together and the Sykes-Moore chamber was partially dismounted so that membrane attached to stroma could be freed from peripheral excess membrane.

Results of transplantation: Control autologous penetrating keratoplasties rapidly thinned to preoperative thickness (Fig. 2). Control penetrating keratoplasties using membranes not seeded with endothelial cells rapidly thicken and remain so indefinitely (Fig. 2). Keratoplasties, in which a membrane seeded with endothelial cells was transplanted, thinned over a 10-12 day period to a thickness comparable to that of the contralateral unoperated eye, and remained so throughout the period of observation which has ranged up to 7 months (Fig. 2).

Normal thickness is attained no more rapidly when Descemet's membrane is removed in addition to native endothelium. However, the technique in which Descemet's, as well as endothelium, is removed is preferred because it is less likely for endothelium on the posterior surface of the membrane to be damaged if the membrane is attached to overlying stroma rather than detached and therefore closer to the iris-lens plane. Eleven of the last fourteen keratoplasties using this technique either with or without the removal of Descemet's in addition to endothelium, have resulted in successes. A success has been considered to occur when the cornea has thinned to normal within a 10-12 day period and remained so throughout the period of observation, including times after which the lids have been occluded to abolish the evaporative effect on corneal thinning. The success rate has also been equally as good whether a relatively thin, 1 μm thick, or relatively thick, 3-5 μm thick, membrane has been used.

At the time of sacrifice, histology has confirmed the presence of morphologically normal endothelium on the posterior surface of the membrane. The origin of the cells as being from tissue culture has been confirmed at

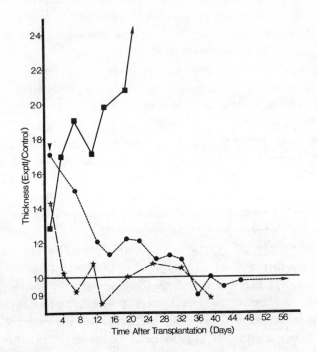

Figure 2 - Graphic representation of corneal thickness of penetrating keratoplasty button relative to corneal thickness of contralateral normal cornea. (·————★————·) autograft in which endothelium is not removed and in which no gelatin membrane or cells from tissue culture are transplanted. (————■————) control stromal autograft with removal of native endothelium and application of gelatin membrane which has not been seeded with tissue cultured corneal endothelial cells. (————●————) stromal autograft after removal of native endothelium and application of gelatin membrane seeded with tissue cultured corneal endothelial cells. (▼) indicates time of apposition of central membrane to overlying stroma.

the time of sacrifice by the presence of scintillation counts of 48-78% of those which were present on the membrane at the time of transplantation.

DISCUSSION

The lack of consistently available donor corneas and the increasing numbers of patients requiring corneal transplantation as the result of endothelial dysfunction, partially secondary to newer techniques in cataract surgery which are more traumatic to corneal endothelium, along with the potential advantages to transplantation of the single layer of endothelial cells, make the development of this technique for man, an attractive one. The successful transplantation of homologous[1-3] and heterologous[5,6] corneal endothelium in animals is encouraging. The principal and still unsolved problem in using these techniques is that of the seeding time of tissue cultured endothelium to autologous stroma. From a surgical standpoint, this technique is an attractive one as it requires no additional surgical skills or alteration in standard penetrating keratoplasty techniques. However, unless the seeding time can be decreased to a 10-15 minute interval, the potential for major complications would seem to outweigh the benefits.

An alternative approach was therefore investigated, as described above, using a thin gelatin membrane as substrate for tissue cultured corneal endothelial cell growth.[4,11] The membrane with cells can be attached to autologous stroma rapidly. In the surgical procedure described, it is possible to attach the membrane to autologous stroma with a time-lapse of 10 minutes from removal of corneal button to replacement of the button with attached membrane and cells back in the recipient bed. The success rate to date has been quite good and is improving as the surgical technique is further refined.

Ideally, the adhesive used should be completely non-toxic. However, it has not been possible as yet to attach the membrane to autologous stroma with a non-toxic adhesive, which is both sufficiently strong and which will last a sufficient period of time to allow the membrane edges to be bound down by scar so that it will not slip. In practice, diluted butylcyanoacrylate has proved to be effective and free of associated complications. Efforts are still being made, however, to find a completely non-toxic adhesive which is sufficiently strong and long-acting.

The other area in need of additional work, before this technique can be applied in man, is in the tissue culture techniques for human corneal endothelium. The most effective tissue culture medium needs to be determined including the most effective and safest growth stimulators or factors. Endeavors are being made along these lines so that human cells may first be transplanted in rabbits, prior to transplantation in lower primates and eventually, in man.

ACKNOWLEDGEMENTS

This work was supported by National Institutes of Health Grant EY-00431.

REFERENCES
1. Maurice, D., McCulley, J., Perlman, M. Donor endothelium from tissue culture. Invest Ophthal, Visual Sci. 16 (ARVO Suppl.):103, 1977 (abst.).
2. Jumblatt, M., Maurice, M., McCulley, J. Transplantation of

tissue-cultured corneal endothelium. Invest Ophthal, Visual Sci. 17:1135-1141, 1978.
3. Maurice, D., McCulley, J., Perlman, M. Development in use of cultured endothelium in corneal transplantation. Docum Ophthal. Proc. Series 20:151-153, 1979.
4. Maurice, D., McCulley, J., Schwartz, B. Keratoplasty with cultured endothelium on thin membranes. Invest Ophthal, Visual Sci. 18(Suppl.):10, 1979 (abst.).
5. Gospodarowicz, D., Greenburg, G., Alvarado, J. Transplantation of cultured bovine corneal endothelial cells to rabbit cornea: Clinical implications for human studies. Proc Natl Acad Sci 76:464-468, 1979.
6. Gospodarowicz, D., Greenburg, G., Alvarado, J. The transplantation in vivo of cultured bovine corneal and vascular endothelial cells in rabbit and cat corneas. Invest Ophthal 18(Suppl):9, 1979 (abst.).
7. Stocker, F.W., Eiring, A., Georgiade, R., and Georgiade, M. A tissue culture technique for growing corneal endothelial, stromal, and endothelial tissue separately. Am J Ophthal 46:294-298, 1958.
8. Lowry, G.M. Corneal endothelium in vitro: Characterization by ultrastructure and histochemistry. Invest Ophthal 5:355-366, 1966.
9. Perlman, M., Baum, J. The mass culture of rabbit corneal endothelial cells. Arch Ophthal 92:235-237, 1974.
10. Baum, J.L., Niedra, R., Davis, C., Yue, B.Y.J.T. Mass culture of human corneal endothelial cells. Arch Ophth 97:1136-1140, 1979.
11. Jumblatt, M., Maurice, D., Schwartz, B. A gelatin membrane substrate for the transplantation of tissue cultured cells. Submitted for publication.

Immunologic protection of corneal allografts

John W.Chandler, M.D.

Corneal Disease Research Laboratory, Eklind Hall, Swedish Hospital Medical Center, 1102 Columbia, Seattle, Washington 98104

ABSTRACT
     Previous work in this laboratory had demonstrated that pretreatment of donor corneas by soaking for 30 minutes in anti-lymphocyte globulin prolonged graft survival and in many cases totally prevented rejections. Follow-up studies seemed to disprove our original hypotheses about the mechanism(s) of immunologic protection, specifically covering up of histocompatibility antigens or production of "enhancing antibody" by the spleen. Recent evidence suggests that our pretreatment reduced or totally eliminated Ia antigen-bearing cells from the cornea and prevented host sensitization. We have been able to produce similar results in mice using high concentrations of oxygen to remove these same cells.

INTRODUCTION

     Corneal allograft refection is currently the major cause of corneal transplant failure [1,2]. In previous work [3-6], we have sought to devise a simple method that would protect corneal allografts from rejection. In all of these studies, we prepared anti-lymphocyte globulin (ALG) by injection of animals with rabbit thymus lymphocytes. The donor corneal allografts were soaked in the ALG for 30 minutes at room temperature. This approach was based on earlier work by Burde and co-workers[7]. They reported that rabbit corneal allografts pretreated with heterologous anti-lymphocyte serum (ALS) had prolonged survival times as compared to unsoaked grafts or grafts pretreated with normal serum. In brief, all of this work demonstrated that corneal allograft refection could be greatly delayed or totally avoided in primary allografts by simple pretreatment with antibody against lymphocytes. However, this pretreatment did not protect the cornea against second-set rejection. We had originally proposed that the antibodies covered up the histocompatibility antigens on corneal allografts and somehow shielded allogeneic graft cells from the host. However, later experiments demonstrated that at least 75 per cent of the antibody was lost by 24 hours and that by six days only a small amount of residual antibody could be detected on the outermost layer of epithelium and on the endothelium. These observations lead us to a consideration of the possibility that antigen-antibody complexes might be shed from the graft and that these might be modulating the immunologic response to the allograft. This hypothesis is based on the observations of Streilin and co-workers [8,9] who demonstrated that allogeneic cells which have been injected into the anterior chamber of rats leave via blood vessels and induce a primary immune response in the spleen. This work suggested that the so-called "immunologic privilege" of the eye is an example of enhancement. Our work, to date, has failed to provide any evidence that this mechanism is operative in our allograft rejection model. We have devoted our recent work to a search for the immunobiological basis for our observations and at the same time have been seeking a simpler method to achieve modification of the graft that would reduce or eliminate corneal graft failure due to allograft rejection. These studies have centered on the possible roll of Ia antigens in host sensitization of corneal allograft recipients and the possibility that pretreatment of donor corneas with ALS or ALG might greatly reduce or eliminate all cells bearing Ia antigen and thereby prolong graft survival or totally prevent host sensitization. Support of such a hypothesis is based on several observations that have recently been published. Ia antigen-bearing cells have been demonstrated in the corneal epithelium of rabbits [10]. These cells have short dendritic processes and may be the equivalent Ia antigen-bearing Langerhans cells in the skin. Studies using inbred guinea pigs are suggestive of a key role for Ia-bearing Langerhans cells in both contact hypersensitivity and skin graft rejection[11]. Finally, antibody to Ia antigens has been detected in ALS [12].

CURRENT RESULTS AND COMMENTS

Our recent work has been devoted to determining the potential role that the elimination of Ia antigen-bearing cells might have played in our model. Ia antigen has been demonstrated in cells of the corneal epithelium of Balb/c and C57/Bl mice as well as strain 2 and strain 13 guinea pigs. These cells have been indentified by indirect fluoresence antibody (F.A.) microscopy using antibody against mouse or guinea pig Ia antigen. These cells tend to have short dendritic processes like those described in rabbits [10]. They are located in the deeper layers of the corneal epithelium especially near the limbus of the cornea. This substantiates the presence of Ia antigen-bearing cells in the cornea.

We have been preparing homologous and heterologous ALG according to our original protocols [3,6]. These will be evaluated for the presence of antibody to Ia antigens. Since Zimmerman et al [12] found such antibody in ALS prepared by immunizing with thymocyte membranes, we are likely to find the same result. Thus, our original work may best be explained by the destruction of Ia-bearing cells in the cornea by ALG and therefore, lack of sensitization of the graft recipient. We have repeated these studies using inbred guinea pigs and intralamellar corneal grafts between strain 2 and 13 animals. The antibody against Ia antigen appears to provide prolonged protection of the allografts against rejection. the pretreatment of corneas with this antibody preparation and complement is associated with few or no Ia-bearing cells when subsequently examined by F.A. The transplant studies have much less convincing. Penetrating keratoplasty is not easily accomplished and we can obtain only a 30-45% rejection rate in our positive controls utilizing intralamellar grafts. Likewise, it is difficult to document the time of onset of rejection in this model. We are currently attempting some different approaches to these technical problems.

Finally, we have been interested in the use of other simple methods to reduce or eliminate Ia antigen-bearing cells from the cornea. Lafferty and co-workers [13] have demonstrated the prolonged survival of endocrine tissue held in organ culture for 12 days in 95 per cent oxygen. We have modified this approach and culture corneas in complete tissue culture medium with 5% dextran (40,000) for 24-48 hours in a hyperbaric chamber at 2 atmospheres of oxygen at 37C. Under these culture conditions, rabbit, guinea pig and mouse cells of the corneal stroma and endothelium survive. The epithelium is largely non-viable and no Ia antigen-bearing cells in mouse or guinea pig corneas can be identified by F.A. Orthotopic corneal grafts in rabbits are easily performed and survive. We have not accumulated enough data in rabbit to prove the beneficial effects of removing Ia antigen-bearing cells.

We have acquired some interesting information in our preliminary mouse studies. The donor corneas were incubated for 24 hours in either 2 atmospheres of oxygen or in 5 per cent CO_2 and room air. Then the donor cornea was placed in subcutaneous tissue in the abdomen. In fresh tissue studies, 100 per cent of corneal grafts from Balb/c into C57/B1 were rejected in 21 days. We have now done several experiments using the pretreated corneas. The table summarizes the results of

Table 1. Incidence of corneal allograft rejection in mice 21 days after transplantation into abdominal wall.

Recipient	Donor-Treatment			
C57/B1	$C57/B1-O_2$	$C57/B1-O_2$	$Balb/c-CO_2$	$Balb/c-O_2$
	0/6*	0/6	5/6	1/6

*Number of grafts rejected
Number of grafts performed

one experiment.

In brief, oxygen treatment appears to modify the donor cornea in some manner and prevent host sensitization and subsequent rejection. Despite the placement of the corneas into subcutaneous sites, unrejected tissue remains clear, non-edematous, and free of infiltration or vascularization. The opposite picture is seen in rejected grafts.

These results need confirmation and extension and such work is in progress in our laboratory. It is tempting to speculate that our original experimental results are best explained by the eduction or total elimination of Ia antigen-bearing cells in the donor corneas. If this can be conclusively proven, then elimination of these cells in donor corneas should lead to a substantial reduction in graft failure due to allograft rejection.

ACKNOWLEDGEMENTS
This work was supported by National Institutes of Health Grant EY-02673

REFERENCES
1. Chandler, J.W., and H.E. Kaufman. 1974. Graft reaction after keratoplasty for keratoconus. Am. J. Ophthalmol. 77:543.
2. Khodadoust, A.A. 1973. The allograft rejection reaction: The leading cause of late failure of clinical corneal grafts. In: Corneal Graft Failure, Ciba Foundation Symposium, Elsevier, Amsterdam, pp. 151.
3. Chandler, J.W, B.M. Gebhardt, and H.E. Kaufman. 1973. Immunologic protection of rabbit corneal allografts: preparation and in vitro testing of heterologous blocking antibody. Invest. Ophthalmol. 12:646.
4. Chandler, J.W., B.M. Gebhardt, J. Sugar, H.E. Kaufman. 1974. Immunologic protection of rabbit corneal allografts: survival of corneas pretreated with succinylated anti-lymphocyte globulin. Transplantation 13:151.
5. Binder, P.S., B.M. Gebhardt, J.W. Chandler, and H.E. Kaufman. 1975. Immunologic protection of rabbit corneal allografts with heterologous blocking antibody. Am. J. Ophthalmol. 79:949.

6. Chandler, J.W. 1976. Immunologic protection of rabbit corneal allografts: prolonged survival of allografts pretreated with homologous antibody against transplantation antigens. Invest. Ophthalmol. 15:213.

7. Burde, R.M., S.R. Waltman, and J.H. Berrios. 1971. Homograft rejection delayed by treatment of donor tissue in vitro with antilymphocyte serum. Science 173:921.

8. Kaplan, H.J., and J.W. Streilin. 1974. Do immunologically privileged sites require a functioning spleen? Nature 251:553.

9. Kaplan, H.J., J.W. Streilin, and T.R. Stevens. 1975. Transplantation immunology of the anterior chamber of the eye. II. Immune response to allogeneic cells. J. Immunol. 115:805.

10. Klareskog, L., U. Forsum, U.M. Tjernlund, L. Rask, and P.A. Peterson. 1979. Expression of Ia antigen-like molecules on cells in the corneal epithelium. Invest. Ophthalmol. 18:310.

11. Stingl, G., S.I. Katz, L. Clement, I. Green, and E.M. Shevach. 1978. Immunologic functions of Ia-bearing epidermal Langerhans cells. J. Immunol. 121:2005.

12. Zimmerman, B., F. Tsui, and T. Delovitch. 1979. Immunosuppressive ALS. II. Antibody to Ia antigens in heterologous anti-lymphocyte serum. Immunol. 37:179.

13. Lafferty, K.J., M.A. Cooley, J. Woolnough, and K.Z. Walker. 1975. Thyroid allograft immunogenicity is reduced after a period in organ culture. Science 188:259.

Host response to allogeneic skin placed in the anterior chamber of the eye

James B.Grogan, Ph.D. and D.S.V.Subba Rao, Ph.D.

Department of Surgery, University of Mississippi Medical Center, 2500 North State Street, Jackson, Mississippi 39216

ABSTRACT

This study was performed to determine the survival time and host immune response to allogeneic skin placed in the anterior chamber of the eye. The results showed that allogeneic Brown Norway skin implants placed in the anterior chamber of Lewis rats survive for several weeks. A positive spleen cell migration inhibition reaction occurs by 14 days post implantation but rejection is not terminated for 6-8 weeks. From 14 to 36 days post implantation, while the implants remain viable, the host demonstrates a period of immunodepression as evidenced by enhancement of orthotopic skin graft survival and a reduced capacity of the host's spleen cells to produce a graft-versus-host response. Serum factors which can block the MIF reaction are detectable in the implant recipient. The presence of the serum factors in the host correlates well with the survival of the implants within the anterior chamber of the eye.

INTRODUCTION

The anterior chamber of the eye is considered to be an immunologically privileged site; however, recent studies have cast some doubt on the true privilege of this site.[1,2,3] It is clear from studies in this laboratory as well as others that tissues are rejected according to their genetic disparity, size, and the type implanted.[1,4] In addition, all tissues are rapidly rejected if the host has been sensitized.[1,5,2] Therefore, the anterior chamber of the eye is privileged under well defined circumstances.[3] There appears to be a delicate control mechanism operative on the host immune system if antigen is presented via the anterior chamber of the eye which determines whether rejection of the allogeneic tissue by immune effector cells will occur or if an active process of immunosuppression occurs which renders the anterior chamber "privileged". The purpose of this study is to show that alloantigen stimulation via the anterior chamber of the eye can transiently produce immunosuppression of host immune system and that serum from viable implant-bearing rats contains factors which are associated with this immuno-suppressive state.

MATERIALS AND METHODS

Experimental animals. Adult rats from Microbiological Associates (Bethesda, MD) and domestically maintained inbred lines of Brown Norway (BN), Fischer (Fi), and Lewis (Le) strains were used in all experiments. Le($Ag-B^1$) rats served as recipients, and donor skin grafts and implants were obtained from BN ($Ag-B^3$) and Fi ($Ag-B^1$) rats.

Skin grafts. Orthotopic skin grafts were transplanted according to the procedure of Billingham[6] with slight modifications as reported by Grogan et al.[7]

Anterior chamber implants. The technique of anterior chamber implanta-tion was essentially that of Medawar[5] as modified by Subba Rao and Grogan.[8] Viability of the implant was evaluated by histological techniques as described previously.[9]

Popliteal lymph node graft-versus-host reaction (GVH). Spleen cells from either normal or implanted rats were prepared as previously described.[10] The resulting cell suspensions were used to perform the popliteal lymph node (PLN) assay developed by Ford et al[11] and modified by Subba Rao and Grogan.[10]

Preparation of test antigens. Antigens were prepared from fresh skin and spleen tissues of BN, Fi, and Le rats as described previously.[8]

Migration inhibition assay. Capillary tubes were filled with a spleen cell suspension (1×10^8/ml), sealed and centrifuged at 500g for 5 minutes. They were cut at the cell fluid interface and were mounted in duplicate in Sykes-Moore chambers with sterile high-vacuum stopcock grease. Capillary tubes from each rat in the experimental and control groups were placed in media containing antigen (0.4 mg/ml) and media containing no antigen. The

chambers were incubated at 37°C for 16-18 hours and the area of cell migration was measured at 30X magnification with a square ocular micrometer. The
cell migration areas were calculated as the number of squares occupied by the
zone of migration.[8] The areas of cell migration of four capillaries
(duplicate chambers) were averaged for each rat, and the percentage of
migration inhibition was calculated by the following formula:

$$\text{percentage of migration} = 1.0 - \frac{\text{area of migration with antigen}}{\text{area of migration with no antigen}} \times 100.$$

Serum blocking tests. Serum was collected from rats bearing implants at
various intervals following implantation. All sera were divided into small
aliquots and were stored at -20°C. Equal volumes of serum and test antigens
were mixed with medium 199 and were used in migration chambers. None of the
sera alone or in combination with antigen caused inhibition of migration of
normal spleen cells.

RESULTS

Immunosuppression in rats bearing viable allogeneic skin implants in the
anterior chamber of the eye. Studies were performed to determine the host
immune response to BN skin implants placed in the anterior chamber of the
eyes of Le rats (Table 1). Rats bearing viable implants for various numbers
of days demonstrated a reduced immune effector system as evidenced by the
delayed rejection of orthotopic skin grafts from the implant donor. Immunosuppression was evident after the implants had been in place for 14 days, but
an even higher degree of immunosuppression was noted in rats that harbored
the implants for 28 days before they received the skin grafts. Skin grafts
applied after 56 days of implant residence, which coincided with the period
when most of the implants were rejected, resulted in a second set rejection
reaction.

Since it appeared that rats bearing viable skin implants in the anterior
chamber of the eye demonstrated the phenomenon of active enhancement, studies
were performed to determine the immune state of the spleen cells from the

Table 1. Immune Response of Lewis Rats Bearing Brown Norway Skin Implants in the Anterior Chamber of the Eye.

| | | Immune Response as Measured by | | |
Days Post Implantation	Implant Viability %	Mean Skin Graft Survival*(Days)	% Migration Inhibition	Graft-versus-Host Response%**
No implants	---	9.4	0	100
7	100	9.6	0	51
14	97	10.8	78	43
21	88	10.9	82	49
28	79	11.4	90	50
42	---	7.5	81	63
56	43	---	76	---
>56	0	7.2	---	90

All groups represented at least 5 animals.

*Skin grafts were applied after the recipient had been implanted in both eyes for the days indicated and the eyes removed at the time of grafting.

**Popliteal lymph node (PLN) enlargement expressed as percent changes in weight of PLN 7 days after footpad injection of 1.0×10^7 spleen cells from Le rats bearing BN implants into F_1 hybrids compared to the weight of the contralateral PLN after injecting a similar number of spleen cells from a normal Le rat. 100% represents the weight of PLN after injection of control spleen cells.

implant-bearing rats. Two in vitro tests were performed: (1) the graft-versus-host reaction and (2) the MIF response. Spleen cells from rats harboring viable implants for 7-35 days exhibited a reduced GVH producing ability as compared to spleen cells from normal rats. Spleen cells from rats bearing long standing implants which were nonviable yielded GVH activity similar to controls but not increased activity as found in skin grafted rats.[10]

The second group of in vitro experiments was performed to determine if the spleen cells from implant-bearing rats exhibited the MIF reaction to alloantigens present on the donor (BN) rat skin. A positive MIF response was evident by 14 days and continued for several weeks even during the period when the host was bearing viable implants and was immunosuppressed.

Blocking of the MIF response with serum from implant-bearing rats. The serum from implant-bearing recipients was investigated to determine if it contained factors which could block the production of lymphokine by syngeneic sensitized spleen cells. Blocking activity was detectable in pooled sera from rats bearing viable implants for 14-28 days (Table 2). The blocking activity of the serum was specific, since neither third party Fischer antigen nor serum from Le rats bearing Fi implants blocked the MIF response produced by the BN implants in the Le rats. Blocking activity was detectable in the rats during the period when most of the implants were viable (Table 3). When rejection

Table 2. Migration of Lewis Spleen Cells in the Presence of Specific Antigen and Sera from Implant-Bearing Rats.

| Group | Migration of Spleen Plus | | % Migration Inhibition |
	Antigen	Serum	
I	None	NRS*	0
II	Brown Norway	None	78
III	Brown Norway	BIS**	+1
IV	Brown Norway	FIS***	72
V	Fischer	None	3

*Normal rat serum - 0.1 ml of normal Lewis rat serum.

**Brown Norway implant serum - 0.1 ml of pooled sera from
   Lewis rats bearing Brown Norway implants for 14-28 days
   was added to the chamber with the antigen.

***Fischer implant serum - 0.1 ml of serum from Lewis rats
   bearing Fischer implant for 14-28 days was added to the
   chamber with the antigen.

Table 3. Correlation Between the Presence of Serum Blocking Activity and Implant Viability in Le Rats Bearing BN Skin Implants in the Anterior Chamber of the Eye.

Weeks Post Implant	% Viable Implants*	% with Blocking Activity**
1	100	0
2	97	78
3	88	87
4	79	94
5	--	24
8	43	0
>8	0	--

*All groups represented at least 5 animals.

**All groups represented at least 12 animals.

of the implants occurred, blocking activity was less often detectable.

DISCUSSION

It has been known for some time that the host can mount an immune response to tissues placed in the anterior chamber of the eye.[9,12,13,14] The present studies show that rats bearing small (0.5 mm^2) fully allogeneic skin implants in the anterior chamber of the eye are immunosuppressed since test skin grafts from the implant donors are significantly prolonged. Other investigators have shown enhancement of skin graft survival in rats injected intracamerally with lymphoid cell suspensions, but a semiallogeneic donor cell population was essential for enhancement to be demonstrated.[15]

Concomitant with the period when the implant recipient exhibited characterization of active enhancement the recipient's spleen cells demonstrated recognition of the donor tissue alloantigens as evidenced by a positive MIF response. However, the GVH response of the spleen cells from these implant recipients indicated a state of immunodepression similar to partial tolerance.[16] It is possible that the antigenic stimulation via the anterior chamber of the eye induces suppressor T cells which results in the reduced GVH reactivity of the spleen cells from the implant-bearing rat. Suppressor T cells have been shown to suppress a number of cell mediated responses including the GVH response.[17,18] When spleen cells from implant-bearing rats were mixed with normal cells, only a slight reduction in the lymph node enlargement was observed.[8] Therefore, our studies were inconclusive about the presence of suppressor cells in this system.

The question that must be asked is how can the host respond with a depressed GVH reaction and a positive MIF reaction at the same time. Obviously these reactions involve different populations of T cells. The MIF response is an indication of early immune recognition by T cells.[19] On the other hand the GVH response is produced by several types of T cells,[20] one of which has effector cell activity[21] and others amplify the reaction.[22]

Observations by Goodnight et al[21] showed that, except in the case of classical neonatal tolerance, hosts bearing organ grafts for long periods of time retain a capacity to respond to donor antigens. The inability of the host to bring about rejection may be due to the production of soluble mediators such as serum blocking factor.[21] These factors could interfere with the maturation process of effector cells after the recognition step.

Guttmann[23] employed the MIF assay to look for blocking factors in enhanced renal allografts. Blocking activity was found 3-5 days after active immunization with spleen cells. The presence of blocking activity did not correlate well with the time of enhancement of kidney allografts.

Using alymphatic skin allografts as privileged sites Merriam and Tilney[24] found an enhancing response with concomitant depression of lymphocyte mediated cytotoxicity, but after 28 days the enhancing effect turned cyto- toxic. Vessella et al[9] showed the presence of cytotoxic lymphocytes in rats bearing large skin implants about the time when most of the implants were rejected or beginning to reject. No attempt was made in that study to detect serum blocking activity.

Even though we have no definite proof that the blocking factor present in the serum of implant-bearing rats bears any relationship to either implant survival or host immunity, it does appear to correlate well with the ability of the implant to·survive in the anterior chamber and with the enhancement of skin graft survival.

ACKNOWLEDGEMENTS

This work was supported in part by U.S.P.H.S. Grant No. AI 09588.

REFERENCES

1. Kaplan, H. J., and T. R. Stevens. 1975. A reconsideration of immunological privilege within the anterior chamber of the eye. Transplantation 19:302.
2. Raju, S., and J. B. Grogan. 1971. Immunology of the anterior chamber of the eye. Transpl. Proc. 3:605.
3. Streilein, J. W., and H. J. Kaplan. 1979. Immunologic privilege in the anterior chamber. In Immunology and Immunopathology of the Eye. Edited by A. M. Silverstein and G. R. O'Connor. Masson, New York. P. 174.
4. Subba Rao, D. S. V., and J. B. Grogan. 1977. Orthotopic skin graft survival in rats which have harbored skin implants in the anterior chamber of the eye. Transplantation 24:377.
5. Medawar, P. B. 1948. Immunity to homologous grafted skin. III. The fate of skin homografts transplanted to the brain, subcutaneous tissue, and to the anterior chamber of the eye. Brit. J. Exptl. Path. 29:58.
6. Billingham, R. E. 1961. Free skin grafting in mammals. In Transplantation of Tissues and Cells. Edited by R. E. Billingham and W. K. Silvers. The Wistar Institute Press, Philadelphia. Pp. 1-23.
7. Grogan, J. B., and B. R. Shivers. 1969. Allograft survival after treatment with antilymphocyte serum combined with immunosuppressive drugs. Surgery 66:1085.
8. Subba Rao, D. S. V., and J. B. Grogan. 1977. Host response to tissues placed in the anterior chamber of the eye: Demonstration of migration inhibition factor and serum blocking activity. Cell. Immunol. 33:125.
9. Vessella, R. L., S. Raju, J. V. Cockrell, and J. B. Grogan. 1978. Host response to allogeneic implants in the anterior chamber of the eye. Invest. Ophthal. Vis. Sci. 17:140.
10. Subba Rao, D. S. V., and J. B. Grogan. 1979. Suppression of graft-versus-host reactions in rats bearing implants in the anterior chamber of the eye. Transplantation 27:75.
11. Ford, W. L., W. Burr, and M. Simonsen. 1970. A lymph node weight assay for the graft-versus-host activity of rat lymphoid cells. Transplantation 10:258.
12. Connelly, D. M. 1961. Transplantation immunity produced by homografts in the anterior chamber. Plastic Reconstruct. Surg. 28:1.

13. Franklin, R. M., and R. A. Prendergast. 1970. Primary rejection of skin allografts in the anterior chamber of the rabbit eye. J. Immunol. 104: 463.

14. Raju, S., and J. B. Grogan. 1969. Heterologous antilymphocyte serum: Influence of immunogenecity on immunosuppressive properties. Transplantation 8:695.

15. Kaplan, H. J., and J. W. Streilein. 1977. Immune response to immunization via the anterior chamber of the eye. I. F1 lymphocyte-induced immune deviation. J. Immunol. 118:809.

16. Heron, J. 1973. Is transplantation tolerance in the rat serum mediated? Transplantation 15:534.

17. Wood, M. L., and A. P. Monaco. Adoptive transfer of specific unresponsiveness to skin allografts by spleen cells from ALS treated, marrow injected mice. Transpl. Proc. 11:1023.

18. Guttmann, R. D. 1977. Mixed leukocyte interaction suppression generated after alloimmunization. Transplantation 24:316.

19. Brondz, B. D., A. P. Suslov, and S. C. Egorova. 1978. Comparative study of cytotoxic T-lymphocytes and producers of the macrophage migration inhibition factor (MIF) in the H-2 system. Scand. J. Immunol. 8:109.

20. Cantor, H., and R. Asofsky. 1970. Synergy among lymphoid cells mediating the graft-versus-host response. II. Synergy in graft-versus-host reactions produced by BALB/c lymphoid cells of differing anatomic origin. J. Exp. Med. 131:235.

21. Goodnight, J. E., D. A. Coleman, and D. Steinmuller. 1976. Serum blocking factors versus specific cellular tolerance in long-term survival of rat heart allografts. Transplantation 22:391.

22. Asofsky, R., H. Cantor, and R. E. Tigelaar. 1971. Cell interactions in the graft-versus-host response. In Progress in Immunology. Edited by B. Amos. Academic Press, New York. P. 369.

23. Guttmann, R. D. 1973. Renal transplantation in the inbred rat. XIX. In vitro correlates of enhancement induction. Transplantation 15:594.

24. Merriam, J. C., and N. L. Tilney. 1978. Prolonged survival of alymphatic skin allografts. A humoral component in the rat. Transplantation 26:87.

Transplantation of corneal endothelium. Allogeneic and xenogeneic transplantation of cell and organ cultures

David BenEzra and Genia Maftzir

The Immuno-Ophthalmology Laboratory, Department of Ophthalmology, Hadassah Hebrew University Hospital, Jerusalem, Israel

ABSTRACT

Thirty-eight surgically successful grafts were performed in 21 rabbits. Allogeneic corneal buttons consisting of epithelium and stroma were kept in culture 48 to 72 hrs and used for transplantation after "repopulation" with rabbit or human cultured endothelial cells or organ Descemet's membranes. Grafts repopulated with organ Descemet's membrane were more successful than those repopulated with endothelial cells only in both the allogeneic and xenogeneic systems. However, while all keratoplasties carried out with corneal buttons repopulated with cultured human endothelial cells failed, repopulation with allogeneic cultured endothelial cells yielded two clear grafts out of six. No hemagglutinating antibodies or in vitro blast transformation of peripheral lymphocytes toward xenogeneic corneal antigens were detected in rabbits that received corneal buttons repopulated by human cultured endothelial cells or organ Descemet's membranes. Transplanting a whole human corneal button induced the appearance of both hemagglutinating antibodies and sensitized lymphocytes towards human and calf corneal antigens.

INTRODUCTION

In humans, transplantation of allogeneic corneas is one of the major ophthalmic surgeries where the success rate is high. While the technical problems have been mastered satisfactorily, the lack of donor material on one hand[1] and the immune graft rejection reactions on the other hand[2] are the remaining obstacles of this rewarding procedure. In order to overcome these stumbling blocks, the idea of corneal preservation in organ culture with a possible lowering of the immunogenicity of the cultured corneas has been investigated[3,4]. In many cases, the refractive disturbance of the cornea is due to endothelial malfunction. In these, the possibility of transplanting only this cellular layer has been recently under consideration in a few laboratories. David Maurice's group advocated the

transplantation of allogeneic cultured corneal endothelial cells
or gelatin membranes[5,6]. Our group was concerned with the
transplantation of an organ endothelial membrane with original
Descemet's in allogeneic and xenogeneic systems in vitro[7].
Denis Gospodarowicz's group made a "more daring" step forward
and suggested the substitution of cultured vascular endothelium
for corneal endothelium[8].

We report herein our in vivo preliminary results on the
transplantation of allogeneic and xenogeneic cultured corneal
endothelial cells and organ Descemet's membranes along with
some observations on specific immune reactions toward the
corneal xenogeneic antigens in these cases.

MATERIALS AND METHODS

Preparation of organ Descemet's membranes: Corneas were
dissected from freshly enucleated rabbit, calf and guinea pig
eyes and from human eyes obtained at autopsy within 24 hours of
death. Descemet's was gently stripped off under the operating
microscope after bathing the corneal button in M-199 (Gibco)
containing antibiotics (penicillin 100 units/ml and streptomicin
100 µg/ml). Great care was taken to avoid any stromal contam-
ination and to obtain a Descemet's membrane without breaks.
After separation from the stroma, Descemet's membrane rolls up
(figure 1a). Flattening of the rolled membrane is carried out
under the microscope with two jewelers forceps. When the membrane is flattened, a drop of M-199 supplemented with 10% calf
serum and antibiotics is added and the plate incubated at $37^{\circ}C$
in an atmosphere of 5% CO_2, 95% air and 100% humidity. Medium
(0.1 ml) containing 10% serum is added daily for five days. On
the sixth day, 2.0 ml of the above medium are added and the
membrane is allowed to float (figure 1b). Endothelial cells
covered both sides of the membrane within two weeks in culture
(figure 1c) and preserved their normal morphology for at least
eight weeks in culture (figure 1d). Before transplantation all
membranes were bathed in medium containing 1% pooled normal
rabbit serum for a few hours.

Cell cultures: These were prepared as previously described[9].
Endothelial cell cultures were initiated from organ Descemet's
membranes of rabbit and human eyes and propagated in cultures
after trypsinization. Stromal and epithelial cells from rabbits

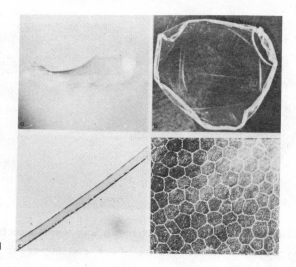

Fig. 1

eyes were prepared similarly[9,10].

Donor corneas: Buttons 11 mm in size were obtained from
freshly enucleated rabbit eyes. Descemet's membrane was removed
from these buttons under the operating microscope and the
remaining epithelium-stroma organ was kept in petri dish (Falcon
3030) with 0.1 ml of M-199 supplemented with 0.1% pooled normal
rabbit serum and incubated as above.

Transplants: These were prepared from the epithelium-
stroma organs according to purpose. For organ Descemet's membrane transplantation, a 7.5 mm trephine button was prepared.
The cultured organ Descemet's membrane was trimmed and sutured
on the button with four sutures of 10-0 nylon (figure 2a and
2b). For endothelial, stromal or epithelial cell transplantation, 10^5 cells in 50 µl were seeded in the center of an 11 mm
freshly prepared corneal button and incubated, as above, for 48
to 72 hours. At the time of keratoplasty, a central 7.5 mm
trephine button was prepared and used as transplant.

Keratoplasty: Albino rabbits of both sexes weighing approximately 3 Kg were used as recipients of the various transplants. Two hours prior to transplantation, Atropine 1% and
scopolamine 0.3% drops were instilled. The rabbits were
sedated by I.V. administration of a solution of pentobarbital
(20 mg/Kg) containing 500 units of heparin. Also, a 300 mg
Aspirin suppository was introduced to the rectum a few minutes

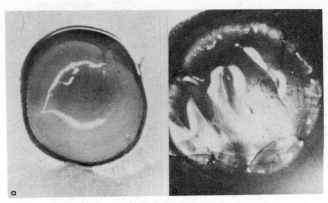

Fig. 2 a

before starting the operation. The eye was then immobilized
with two stay-sutures under the inferior and superior recti. A
7.0 mm corneal button from the host cornea was removed by
trephine and corneal scissors. During the operation, the eye
was constantly irrigated with 0.5% neomycin solution. After
removal of the host button, the 7.5 mm donor button was secured
with 12 to 16 separated 8-0 nylon sutures. In some cases, the
lens was extracted and anterior vitrectomy performed before
suturing of the graft. Twenty-four hours after grafting,
freezing of the remaining host cornea was carried out by two
sets of 10 second applications with a cryoprobe destroying most
of the host endothelial cells.

Post operative treatment: At the end of surgery, a subconjunctival injection of 2 mg Depomedrol, atropine 1% drops, syn-
thomycetin eye ointment and an intramuscular injection of 500,000
units of penicillin G were given. Apart from the Depomedrol
injection, the above treatment was continued for seven days.
One week after surgery, the penicillin injections were stopped
and the local treatment continued for four weeks.

Evaluation of the graft: Daily observations of the grafts
were carried out under the microscope and slit lamp. Clarity of
the graft was arbitrarily scored according to the possibility of
observing the ocular structures behind the graft. Thus, (+++)
denotes an opaque graft, (++) a very edematous graft, (+) edematous graft, (+) indicates a hazy graft and (-) a clear non-
edematous graft without any flare reaction in the anterior chamber.

Immune parameters: Four weeks. after transplantation, blood from the marginal ear was withdrawn from the graft recipients. Antibodies to allogeneic and xenogeneic corneas were tested using the indirect hemagglutination technique[11], while cellular sensitivity was tested by the blast transformation of lympho- cytes on re-exposure to the various corneal antigens in vitro[12].

RESULTS

Morphology of the transplant in its side facing the anterior chamber: The bare stromal surface of the cultured corneal button is shown in figure 3a. The collagen fibers are thicker than normal. The additional photographs in figure 3 demonstrate the appearance 48 hours after seeding of cultured rabbit endothelial cells (3b), keratocytes (3c), or epithelial cells (3d). Cultured human corneal cells seeded on the rabbit corneal buttons, adhered to the "bare" rabbit stroma but showed a lack of uniformity (figure 4a). The endothelial cells on the organ cultured Descemet's membrane, on the other hand, showed a more preserved morphology (figure 4b).

Fate of grafts: Table 1 demonstrates the various proced- ures, operative complications and the condition of the grafts 24 hours after surgery. Due to the incubation of the allogeneic buttons, all grafts were very edematous before transplantation to recipients. At the end of surgery, following suture tight- ening, the grafts became less edematous. All grafts derived from cultured buttons were less edematous 24 to 72 hours after transplantation than before their grafting into recipient beds. Thirty-eight technically successful experimental grafts were performed in 21 rabbits. Fifteen grafts were repopulated with allogeneic endothelial, stromal or epithelial cells and allo- geneic organ Descemet's membranes; eleven grafts were repopu- lated with xenogeneic endothelial cells or organ Descemet's membranes, and twelve grafts were used as controls (Table 1).

Of the grafts repopulated with allogeneic cells, four were with an organ Descemet's membrane, three were repopulated with stromal cells, two with epithelial cells, and six with endothelial cells (Table 2). Of the four grafts with cultured Descemet's membrane, two were clear and without any reaction in the anterior chamber; one graft was slightly hazy with a mild

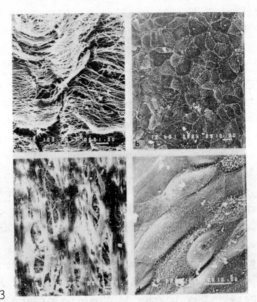

Fig. 3

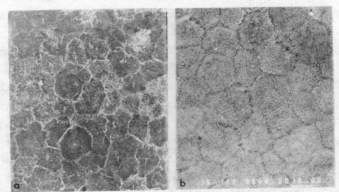

Fig. 4

Table 1:   Treatment and operative complications in 21 rabbits

Rabbit	Eye	Treatment	Operative complications	Edema of graft [5]
1	OD	R.Dm.	Removal of lens and vitrectomy	++
	OS	--	Not operated	-
2 [1]	OD	Sham op.	None	-
	OS	Ep-St.	None	-
3	OD	H.En.	None	++
	OS	H.En.	Anterior synechiae	++
4	OD	R.En.	None	+
	OS	R.En.	None	++
5	OD	R.St.	Technical failure	++
	OS	R.St.	None	+
6	OD	R.Ep.	None	++
	OS	R.Ep.	Removal of lens and vitrectomy	++
7	OD	H.En.	None	++
	OS	H.En.	None	+
8 [2]	OD	Ep-St.	None	+
	OS	Ep-St.	None	++
9	OD	R.Dm.	None	+
	OS	R.Dm.	None	+
10	OD	H.Dm.	Removal of lens and vitrectomy	++
	OS	H.En.	Technical failure	++
11	OD	Cryo [3]	None	±
	OS	R.En.	None	++
12	OD	H.C.	None	++
	OS	H.C.	None	++
13	OD	R.St.	None	++
	OS	R.Dm.	None	++
14	OD	R.St.	None	++
	OS	R.En.	None	++

Table 1 - continued

Rabbit	Eye	Treatment	Operative complications	Edema of (5) graft
15	OD	H.Dm.	None	+
	OS	H.Dm.	None	++
16	OD	Cryo (4)	None	±
	OS	--	Not operated	-
17	OD	H.C.	None	++
	OS	H.C.	None	++
18	OD	R.En.	None	++
	OS	R.En.	None	++
19	OD	R.C.	None	±
	OS	R.C.	Anterior synechiae	+
20	OD	R.C.	None	+
	OS	R.C.	None	+
21	OD	R.C.	None	+
	OS	R.C.	None	+

Legends to Table 1:
(1) Autologous transplantation without in vitro incubation of the grafts.
(2) Allogeneic transplantation after in vitro incubation of the grafts for 48 hours.
(3) Cryo applications were performed on the whole cornea including the central 7 mm of the graft.
(4) Cryo applications were performed on the recipient corneal area avoiding the central 7 mm of the graft.
(5) Assessed 24 hours after surgery. (-) denotes clear graft without reaction in the anterior chamber; (±), slightly hazy graft accompanied with mild flare in the anterior chamber; (+), edematous graft with marked flare in the anterior chamber; (++), very edematous graft, structures in the anterior chamber are barely seen; (+++), opaque graft, structure in the anterior chamber not seen.
R=rabbit; H=human; Dm.=cultured organ Descemet's membrane; En.= cultured endothelial cells; Ep-St.=non repopulated graft consisting of epithelium and stroma only; H.C.=cultured human cornea including all layers; R.C.=cultured rabbit cornea including all layers.

flare in the anterior chamber, and one graft remained slightly edematous four weeks after surgery. Among the three grafts repopulated with stromal cells, two were very edematous and opacified while one graft started to show less edema the third week after surgery. The two eyes repopulated with epithelial cells showed the highest degree of opacification already apparent after the first week. Of the six buttons repopulated with cultured endothelial cells, one was completely clear without any reaction in the anterior chamber and one graft was slightly hazy and accompanied by a mild flare in the anterior chamber. Two grafts were very edematous and opacified while two others improved slightly but remained edematous four weeks after surgery (Table 2).

Whole human corneal grafts resulted in very edematous

Table 2: Fate of grafts repopulated with allogeneic cells

Rabbit	Eye	Treatment	Edema of graft on follow-up			
			24 hrs	1 week	2 weeks	4 weeks
1	OD	R.Dm.	++	+	$\pm$	-
4	OD	R.En.	+	++	+	$\pm$
	OS	R.En.	++	++	+	++
5	OS	R.St.	+	++	++	$\pm$
6	OD	R.Ep.	++	+++	+++	+++
	OS	R.Ep.	++	++	++	+++
9	OD	R.Dm.	$\pm$	+	$\pm$	-
	OS	R.Dm.	+	++	+	$\pm$
11	OS	R.En.	++	+	+	+
13	OD	R.St.	++	++	+++	+++
	OS	R.Dm.	++	+	$\pm$	+
14	OD	R.St.	++	+	++	++
	OS	R.En.	++	+	++	++
18	OD	R.En.	++	+	++	+
	OS	R.En.	++	+	+	-

For legend, see Table 1.

opaque and vascularized grafts in all four cases (Table 3).
Repopulation of the allogeneic buttons with cultured human
endothelial cells slightly improved the fate of the grafts.
Two of these remained very edematous and opacified. One graft
demonstrated slight improvement on longer follow-up and became
only slightly edematous three weeks after surgery. One graft
improved markedly and four weeks after surgery showed a mild
flare in the anterior chamber and a slightly hazy graft. Transplanting a whole Descemet's membrane appeared to improve the
fate of the graft repopulated with xenogeneic endothelial cells.
One of these became completely clear without any reaction in
the anterior chamber, one remained slightly hazy with a mild
flare in the anterior chamber, while the third graft remained
edematous and opacified (Table 3).

The control grafts consisted of one sham operation that
remained clear throughout the period of study. One autologous
graft, from which Descemet's membrane and endothelium were
removed, opacified. Two allogeneic grafts devoid of Descemet's
membrane and endothelium that were kept in culture before

Table 3: Fate of grafts repopulated with xenogeneic (human)
endothelial cells, organ Descemet's membrane or whole cornea

			Edema of graft on follow-up			
Rabbit	Eye	Treatment	24 hrs	1 week	2 weeks	4 weeks
3	OD	H.En.	++	++	+	±
	OS	H.En.	++	++	++	++
7	OD	H.En.	++	++	++	++
	OS	H.En.	+	++	+	+
10	OD	H.Dm.	++	++	±	-
12	OD	H.C.	+	++	+++	+++
	OS	H.C.	++	++	+++	+++
15	OD	H.Dm.	+	++	++	+
	OS	H.Dm.	++	++	+	±
17	OD	H.C.	+	+++	+++	+++
	OS	H.C.	+	+++	+++	+++

For legend, see Table 1.

keratoplasty remained edematous throughout. Two autologous grafts served as controls for the cryo applications. One of these received applications over the whole cornea and opacified; the other received cryo applications over the recipient bed only, avoiding the central 7 mm area, and remained clear throughout. Six cultured rabbit whole corneas that were grafted thinned gradually and were all clear the fourth week after surgery (Table 4). None of these eyes showed any reaction in the anterior chamber on last examination.

Immune studies: There were no detectable immune responses toward the corneal antigens after repopulation of the corneal buttons with allogeneic or xenogeneic cultured endothelial cells or organ Descemet's membranes. Hemagglutinating antibodies against human and calf corneal antigens as well as a weak specific blast transformation reaction against these antigens were found in the two rabbits that were grafted with cultured whole human corneal grafts (Table 5). A hemagglutinating titer of 1/8 with a borderline significant blast transformation reaction

Table 4: Fate of control grafts

Edema of graft on follow-up

Rabbit	Eye	Treatment	24 hrs	1 week	2 weeks	4 weeks
2[2]	OD	Sham op.	±	−	−	−
	OS	Ep-St.	−	+	++	++
8[2]	OD	Ep-St.	+	++	+++	+++
	OS	Ep-St.	++	++	+++	+++
11[3]	OD	Cryo	±	+	++	+
16[4]	OD	Cryo	±	−	−	−
19	OD	R.C.	±	±	−	−
	OS	R.C.	+	±	−	−
20	OD	R.C.	+	±	−	−
	OS	R.C.	+	±	±	−
21	OD	R.C.	+	−	−	−
	OS	R.C.	+	±	−	−

For legend, see Table 1.

was also detected against calf corneal antigens in rabbit 19
receiving cultured whole rabbit corneas (Table 5).

DISCUSSION

Due to the limited number of grafts studied, definite
conclusions are deferred until data from additional experiments
now in progress will be available. Nevertheless, from the

Table 5: Immune responses of recipient toward allogeneic and
xenogeneic ocular antigens

Humoral and cellular immune responses[*]

Rabbit	Transplant	Fate of grafts	Hemagglutination			Blast transformation		
			R.C.	H.C.	C.C.	R.C.	H.C.	C.C.
2	Auto-logous	clear clear	0	0	4[1]	1.0[2]	1.2	1.8
3	H.En.	hazy opaque	0	0	0	0.8	1.6	0.9
7	H.En.	opaque edema	0	0	0	1.3	1.0	2.1
9	R.Dm.	clear hazy	0	0	4	1.2	0.6	0.8
12	H.C.	opaque opaque	2	16	16	0.9	4.2	3.1
15	H.Dm.	opaque hazy	0	0	0	1.4	1.6	1.2
17	H.C.	opaque opaque	2	32	8	1.3	2.8	2.0
18	R.En.	edema clear	0	0	0	1.0	0.7	1.5
19	R.C.	clear clear	0	0	8	1.2	1.7	2.8

* Performed 4 weeks after surgery.
(1) indicates the reciprocal highest dilution of serum giving
positive hemagglutination. 0 = no hemagglutination of a serum
dilution of 1/2.
(2) index of stimulation = H^3 Thymidine uptake with stimulated
antigen/H^3 Thymidine in control cultures.

reported results of this study it appears that transplantation of allogeneic cultured endothelial cells or organ Descemet's membranes can be successful. Moreover, xenogeneic transplantation of cultured corneal endothelial cells and to a greater extent cultured xenogeneic organ Descemet's membranes, may show some success. At least the immune reactions toward the xenogeneic transplanted cultured endothelial and organ Descemet's membranes seem to be negligible as compared to immune responses observed when transplantation is performed with cultured whole xenogeneic corneas[3,4] and as shown in this study.

Apart from the better performance of the cultured organ Descemet's membranes as compared to the cultured endothelial cells in both the allogeneic and xenogeneic systems as observed in this study, additional advantages of the organ Descemet's membranes can be expected: First, there is an assurance that a whole sheet of healthy and active endothelial cells is transplanted. Second, due to the fact that the Descemet's membrane can be sutured on the graft during the keratoplasty, an autologous transplantation of the epithelial and stromal layers could be possible.

The possibility of transplanting only one crucial cellular layer and obtaining a successful graft is of great practical application in ophthalmology. This approach could open a new era in transplantation surgery on one hand, and in transplantation immunity on the other hand. The results thus far are encouraging and very promising; however, more experiments and longer follow-up are needed. Also, endothelial cells or organ Descemet's membrane xenografting in primates is necessary before any conclusions for applications in humans can be drawn.

ACKNOWLEDGEMENTS

We are thankful to Mr. A. Zelikovitch for the preparation of the photographs and to Ms. J. Fisher and H. Gnessin for their help in preparing the manuscript.

REFERENCES

1. Chirambo, M.C., and D. BenEzra. 1976. Causes of blindness among students in blind school institutions in a developing country. Brit. J. Ophthalmol. 60: 665.
2. Khodadoust, A.A. 1973. The allograft rejection reaction. The leading cause of late failure of clinical corneal grafts.

In Corneal Graft Failure, Ciba Foundation Symposium, p. 151. Elsevier, Amsterdam.

3. BenEzra, D., and U. Sachs. 1975. Growth and transplantation of organ cultured corneas. Invest. Ophthalmol. 14: 24.

4. Doughman, D.J., G.E. Miller, E.A. Mindrup, and J.E. Harris. 1976. The fate of experimental organ-cultured corneal xenografts. Transplantation 22: 132.

5. Jumblatt, M.M., D.M. Maurice, and J.P. McCulley. 1978. Transplantation of tissue cultured corneal endothelium. Invest. Ophthalmol. Vis. Sci. 17: 1135.

6. Maurice, D.M., J.P. McCulley, and B.D. Schwartz. 1979. Keratoplasty with cultured endothelium on thin membranes. Invest. Ophthalmol. Vis. Sci. 18 (ARVO Suppl.): 10.

7. BenEzra, D. 1978. Transplantation of endothelial membrane. An in vitro study. Invest. Ophthalmol. Vis. Sci. 17 (ARVO Suppl.): 253.

8. Gospodarowicz, D., G. Greenburg, and J. Alvarado. 1978. Transplantation of cultured bovine corneal endothelial cells to rabbit cornea: clinical implications for human studies. Proc. Nat. Acad. Sci. 76: 464.

9. BenEzra, D. 1977. A microculture technique for the evaluation of corneal cell metabolism in vitro. Invest. Ophthalmol. 16: 893.

10. BenEzra, D., and T. Tanishima. 1978. Possible regulatory mechanism of the cornea. I. Epithelial-stromal interaction in vitro. Arch. Ophthalmol. 96: 1891.

11. Gery, I. and A.M. Davies. 1961. Organ specificity of the heart. I. Animal immunization with heterologous heart. J. Immunol. 87: 351.

12. BenEzra, D. 1976. Experimental specific memory reactions to cornea, lens and retina antigens. Arch. Ophthalmol. 94: 661.

SESSION IV

Summary of Discussion

In the discussion on ocular tumor immunology the question arose of antigenic similarity of ocular melanomas to those which may develop at other sites. While cross reactivity of melanoma associated antigens in human skin and choroidal tissue exist, there is a paucity of available tumor material from choroidal melanomas to allow for generation of sufficient data on the specificity of humoral reactivity to the antigens. Additionally, biologic features of choroidal and skin malanomas vary both in terms of malignant potential and metastatic pattern.

It was agreed that assessment on the differentiation of orbital pseudotumor from lymphoma may be difficult, with histopathologic diagnosis carrying an error rate of up to 40 percent. However, immunohistologic techniques may be more useful although their efficacy in orbital tumor diagnosis remains unproven. While in most cases pseudotumors appear heterogeneous and lymphomas monoclonal in their respective immunologic characterizations, this is not always so. On occasion patients with lymphoma appear to bear polyclonal tumors and some with benign disease do have monoclonal proliferation. It is expected that the use of hybridoma produced monoclonal antibodies may improve the accuracy of this diagnostic technique.

Data could not be offered on the role of NK cells in tumor resistance. However, it was indicated that since engraftment tumor is often related to the number of implanted cells with resistance observed at low dose levels, it would seem reasonable to suppose that resistance in part may be due to the local presence of natural cytotoxic cells. Regarding thymus leukemic antigen (TLA) associated tumor killing, the necesary formal genetic experiments to evaluate this concept have not yet been performed. However, in early work two loci appear to have been detected. One is in or close to TLA but without correlation to any of the Qa determinants; the other is unrelated to TLA and seemingly derived from the A background in mice.

In discussions on the immunobiology of the cornea, it was pointed out that Ia skin antigens, once believed to be located on keratinocytes, are in fact located only on Langerhans cells; these represent approximately 3-5 percent of cells within the epidermis. A relevant recent report has confirmed the belief of absence of Langerhans cells and Ia antigens in the cornea[1]. Nevertheless, the indication is that the absence of Ia antigens from corneal epithelium is still not universally accepted (positive findings by Kleriskog[2]) although it is agreed that their absence from endothelium and stroma seems likely.

Pertinent also is the absence of mast cells in the cornea and the belief that "passenger" leucocytes are not involved in corneal rejection. Thus, few if any leucocytes may be found in corneal tissue. From an experimental standpoint, a corneal implant may remain under favorable conditions for a period of as long as a year, and then when retransplanted to an appropriate recipient will again display all of the initial properties of a correspondingly early transplant.

Discussion was next directed to the point that corneal graft rejection may not necessarily involve presently known Ia antigens. An example of this is the presence of T cell associated Ia antigens (on both suppressor and helper cells) in other tissues that are absent on B cells, suggesting the possibility that Ia antigens which are as yet serologically undefined may be providing the antigenic stimulus in the cornea. Additionally, serologic definition of Ia antigens may be inadequate in providing the full range of T lymphocyte recognition. Thus, it was noted that Ia positive cells which lack LD fail to stimulate T helper cells, inviting the question as to whether cells from any of the corneal layers do have LD antigens which may activate Ly 1 T helper cells. In commenting on this point it was noted that although this information is not presently known, it is quite possible to devise such investigations since cells from various corneal layers can feasibly be cultured.

The suggestion was offered that Qa antigens may play some role in raising the cellular immune response level to allogeneic cells and corneal graft rejection. In this regard the development of immunity and killer cells against Qa 1 antigen was cited; also the fact that Ia can help with Qa recognition. Finally, it was pointed out that corneal cells do stimulate allogeneic lymphocyte proliferation in vitro.

Agreement was expressed with the concept that corneal cells act immunologically in the same fashion as other cells, yet data were cited on GVH reactions in lymphocyte transfers where ocular tissues are usually spared in responding animals. In further discussion of distinctions between corneal and skin grafts which centered on two presumed differences, i.e., cell type and privileged site, the position taken was that the principal distinguishing factor involves site privilege. Skin implanted on cornea will not act differently from cornea itself; cornea implanted ectopically will not act differently from skin with respect to sensitization and rejection. Additionally, it was noted that even when neovascularization occurs in the cornea its physiologic environment resembles the skin only in part; vascularization occurs slowly and incompletely so that access to the lymphatic system remains poor.

Discussion was entered into the role of HLA in keratoplasty. Here it was reported that human corneal allografts are rejected less often when transplanted into human hosts if the hosts lack preformed antibodies against donor histocompatibility antigen, i.e., negative cross matching. On the other hand, no benefit has been found when there is HLA similarity of donor and host. In extended discussion, the importance of DR (Ia mouse equivalent) antigens in the human in allograft rejection was emphasized.

The suggestion was then offered that recipient suppressor T cells induced by donor corneal cells following preparation in tissue culture might be placed in the eye at the time of the graft or when the rejection process begins. If necessary, such cells could be stored by established cryopreservation techniques until such time as needed. The question of possible correlation between corneal graft rejection and blood groups was answered by the lack of demonstrable effect in mismatches. Additionally, it was noted that studies in experimental animals support the concept that D antigens are important in rejection phenomena; this work should provide guidance on issues to be addressed.

Attention was then given to consideration of the fact that three significant factors in advancing the art of corneal transplantation had little to do with immunology: (1) application of techniques made possible by the use of the surgical microscope, (2) development of better sutures to reduce neovascularization, and (3) use of topical corticosteroids. Since vascularization appears essential to the problem of corneal rejection, a possibility was raised concerning pretreatment of recipients locally with either antibody or cells directed against differentiation antigens found on blood vessels in order to preempt vascularization by producing vessel necrosis. In further considering the suggestion that angiogenesis growth factor might be involved in vascularization, other possible mechanisms for the maintenance and/or modification of the normal state should be investigated, e.g., antiangiogenesis growth factor antibody as a controlling factor.

Especially pertinent may be the point that the principal existing clinical problem concerns patients whose corneas have become vascularized and who are at the same time hyperimmunized. In normal surgery, vascularization is unlikely unless there is coincident development of an abscess or an ulcer. Even then, rejection may not occur until the graft is further irritated, e.g., by suture removal. Again, a long term successful implant may be rejected following rejection from the other eye in a later implant.

Information is not available on whether anterior chamber aqueous from an eye undergoing corneal graft rejection would induce neovascularization if placed in a normal eye. However, the existence of a factor in normal rabbit aqueous which inhibits neovascularization has been reported. Further, caution was expressed that any process developed to reduce neovascularization must not affect limbal vasculature in order that the cornea not become completely ischemic. Also, it was pointed out that it is in only the small proportion of cases where corneal grafts are repeatedly rejected that clinicians are in need of the type of help that can be offered by immunologic approaches. Finally, it was emphasized that the cornea could provide an ideal system for studying human transplantation immunology and technology since two important elements exist, corneal cells can be cultured and healthy recipients are readily available.

Inquiry was made into the applicability of methods for cultivating vascular endothelium to corneal endothelial cell culture. In describing approaches based upon the use of an extracellular matrix, it was noted that most cells that failed to grow in tissue culture did not produce a suitable extracellular matrix and further that polystryrene tray surfaces are inadequate. Accordingly, a successful technique involves the growing of a cell monolayer which produces a matrix, removal of the cells with triton X, and then subsequent culturing of corneal or vascular endothelial cells on the remaining matrix. Regarding the nature of similarities between vascular and corneal endothelial cells, further observation was offered that although these may not be the same, they do function physiologically in the same manner when located on the back of the cornea.

The issue of immunization of corneal graft recipients was then addressed. In experimental studies involving the rat, epidermal cells placed in the anterior chamber sensitize an allogeneic recipient; however, data are not available with cell numbers smaller than 5×10^5, and the nature of this immunologic response appears to be different from that obtained by sensitization of other sites.

In noting that non-viable stroma is not antigeneic and not rejected, the question of its transparency arose. Indications are that dead stroma may remain clear when layered on healthy endothelium and further, that while such stroma produces inflammation in xenogeneic tissues, rarely does this happen in allogeneic tissue.

In discussing post-responses to allogeneic skin placed in the anterior chamber of the eye, it was felt important to emphasize the unique anatomical situation of the anterior chamber that allows for absence of lymphatic drainage and the direct access of all released antigens to the blood circulation. While this factor could lead to poor immune responses to antigens released into the anterior chamber, it was noted that the anterior chamber is a privileged site only under very specific conditions, and that xenogeneic tissues never survive these at all. Additionally relevant is the fact that all implants become vascularized and infiltrated with mononuclear cells within 10-14 days.

Transplantation of cultured corneal endothelial tissue was then discussed. Emphasized was the importance of the application of cultured corneal endothelial cells as an autograft, particularly when corneal regrafting is required, suggesting that extensions of such techniques to the use of autologous venous endothelium could be of great value. Especially

to be sought would be the application of endothelial transplantation in

Fuchs' dystrophy and dystrophy of the endothelium.

REFERENCES

1. Streilein, J. W., G. B. Toews and P. R. Bergstresser. 1979. Corneal
allografts fail to express Ia antigens. Nature 282:326.
2. Klareskog, L., U. Forsum, U. Malmnas-Tjernlund, L. Rask and P. A.
Peterson. 1979. Expression of Ia antigen-like molecules on cells in the
corneal epithelium. Invest. opthalmol. 18:310.

SESSION V

Assessments and recommendations for future vision research

Prepared by the Moderators: F.Bach and H.Cantor

Having considered immunogenetic aspects of corneal transplantation and eye tumors, and immune disorders relevant to the eye and ocular infectious processes during this meeting, the panel was able to offer a set of pertinent recommendations that follow.

Of central importance was the development of interdisciplinary approaches involving immunogeneticists, immunobiologists and experts in ophthalmic disease. For such endeavors, the panel believed that each of the areas considered below represents a field of investigation feasible to approach at the present time. Additionally, it was felt that the results of such investigation could be expected to contribute to the further understanding of fundamental biological processes and further our understanding of these subjects as they apply to human disease. Within the group of potentially productive areas for investigation, an assignment of priorities was found to be difficult. However, in the list that follows, an attempt has been made to rank items in some order of importance, based to a considerable extent on the degree of attention attracted during this workshop. In each of the areas mentioned, the panel felt strongly that wherever possible studies in experimental animal models would be required as well as the conduct of clinical investigation in man.

It was suggested in the strongest terms that mechanisms be found to train and attract immunogeneticists and immunobiologists to departments of

ophthalmology to engage in an active manner initially in the specific
research areas mentioned and subsequently in others as they are developed.
It was the feeling of the group that collaborative efforts between individuals in different departments would be useful, but that such collaborative
efforts would not serve as effectively as those involving immunologically
trained scientists totally immersed in eye disease research. Such training
programs should include both individuals dedicated to working in human
diseases and veterinarians for the study of animal diseases relevant to
problems in man.

Immunological Problems Relating to Transplantation of the Cornea

Major emphasis should be given to defining the various antigens
present on different cell types of the cornea including those of the
epithelial, stromal and endothelial layers. The character of eye tissue
antigens should be studied with the use of specific antisera, including
monoclonally derived reagents, and also by cellular techniques such as
mixed leucocyte cultures (MLC) and primed LD typing (PLT). It will be of
particular interest to determine whether all identifiable types of antigens
encoded by the major histocompatibility complex (MHC), including the
homologues of I region and K/D region encoded antigens, are present on the
various cells. This problem can be best approached by using those available
serologic reagents known to detect the antigens of one or another type or
through the use of cell mediated immune systems with cells generated in
mixed leukocyte culture. In addition to experiments designed to evaluate
the presence of MHC encoded antigens on corneal cells, attempts should be
made to define possible tissue specific antigens both by production of
monoclonal reagents as well as by transplantation techniques.

Investigations designed to define the arms of the immune response that
participate in corneal rejection should be encouraged. The investigations
should include probing of both cell mediated and antibody mediated mechanisms

in both primary and second set graft rejection. Continued typing for the
HLA-A, -B, -C, and -D antigens is recommended; also emphasized is the
importance of cross-matching potential recipients for the presence of
antibodies against antigens in donor cornea. Although there is evidence at
present suggesting a correlation between HLA typing, cross-matching and
improved graft survival, this correlation is not conclusive. Hence, as a
part of these studies, retrospective evaluation of the influence of such
factors as prior blood transfusions, age and sex should be included.

HLA and Disease

A number of different disorders of the eye should be evaluated for
possible associations between HLA antigens and the diseases in question.
It would seem wise to focus on those disorders where there appears to be
heterogeneity of the disease entity based on clinical evaluation. As a
part of these studies, epidemiologic investigation concerned with location,
prevalence, and the role of the environment in these diseases should be
pursued.

Pseudo-tumors and Lymphomas of the Eye

The types of cells present in pseudo-tumors and lymphomas of the eye
should be characterized. Reagents that will distinguish T and B lymphocytes,
null and NK cells as well as various subpopulations of T lymphocytes should
be employed. In addition, studies of cell functions should be pursued,
i.e., to define helper, cytotoxic or suppressor status with regard to
T lymphocytes and to determine if the tumors are monoclonal.

Studies in Autoimmunity and Infectious Diseases of the Eye

With regard to infectious diseases of the eye, emphasis on herpes
simplex keratouveitis is indicated in an attempt to understand the basis of
potential immune reactions to the herpes virus in associative recognition
with self histocompatibility antigens. Also an analysis of the possible
associations between HLA antigens and susceptibility to herpes keratouveitis

and certain other eye disease entities is worthy of study.

Definition of the antigenic moieties that are recognized by the organism and that evoke a response in autoimmune disorders, as found in experimental retinitis, is highly important to provide leads for extending investigation of these diseases.

Studies of genetic control of autoimmune reactions against ocular components, both in experimental animals and in man, is also recommended. In addition, recently introduced approaches based on immunogenetic knowledge should be applied to the modulation of ocular autoimmune disease, e.g., those involving anti-idiotype immunity, and antibodies against certain MHC antigens, etc.

Included in the above recommendations are representative examples that should be extended to other infections and autoimmune reactions that occur in the eye. It is anticipated that some of these topics will be dealt with more extensively during the subsequently planned National Eye Institute immunology workshops.

Afterword

Arthur M.Silverstein

It is the usual practice of a conference summarizer to go through the
table of contents of the volume, rehearsing one by one the names of the
authors, the subject of their presentations, and perhaps a highlight or
two from each manuscript. But the interested reader can obtain this for
himself from this volume, and in any event it is often true at symposiums
that what is said in the formal sessions is of less long-term significance
than are the discussions and collaborations that develop outside of the
meeting room -- during coffee breaks, in the hallways, in the dining room,
and during late-night heated discussions in the cocktail lounge. In order
to tell this part of the conference story, your normally sober and abstem-
ious reporter spent most of his off-hours circulating from one group to
another with ears wide open, drinking too much coffee, eating too much food,
raising his blood-alcohol level to unusual heights, but willingly paying
this high price for the information obtained.

As is often the case when specialists from two very disparate fields meet
together, total confusion reigned at the start. The basic immunologists
left the ophthalmologists dazed with their talk of isotypes and idiotypes;
of T-cell subsets with their confusing congeries of surface markers; and
of complicated interacting networks of suppressor cells and enhancer cells.
The ophthalmologists, in their turn, quite baffled immunologists with their

talk of clinical keratoplasty employing grafts which, while immunologically "privileged", could be rejected; with the confusing array of anterior and posterior diseases known by the collective but not very enlightening term uveitis; and with the fact that good models of most human eye diseases do not exist in the mouse (the species with which immunologists are most comfortable, and in which they have been able minutely to dissect complicated mechanisms and to define much of modern immunology). The early confusion was such that the members of each speciality huddled protectively with one another, asking, "Who are these strangers? What in God's name are they talking about?" and "Why are we here?".

Slowly, however, small signs developed that communication was starting between the two groups, so that as early as breakfast-time on the second day, immunologists and ophthalmologists could be seen mixing at the same table, and an immunologist was even overhead to say to an ophthalmologist, "That's very interesting! Tell me more about ...", while an ophthalmologist startled his neighbours by saying, "I wonder whether I couldn't use your clone of Ly 1, 2 lymphocytes to ...". As the conference continued, there was an almost palpable increase in the interdisciplinary interactions, so that by the time the meeting ended most conferees could express pleasant surprise at what they had learned about the other discipline, and many left excited by new research ideas.

It would be impossible to detail all of the accomplishments of this symposium, since some will undoubtedly be delayed by the time that it may take for the germ of an idea planted during the conference to sprout and grow into a formal experiment or research project. Nevertheless, we can list a number of useful consequences of the meeting. First, the ophthalmic members of the group were clearly impressed by the precision with which immunologic mechanisms are being dissected, and by the techniques and reagents at the command of the immunologist. Already at the meeting, interdisciplinary deals and collaborations were being negotiated, to search for new membrane antigens that might be important for corneal graft rejection; to utilize lymphocyte clones to study mechanisms of target cell destruction and immunoregulation in ocular disease; to study the role of H-region genes in viral infections; and to apply the latest knowledge of immunogenetics to improve prognosis in keratoplasty and to better understand the basis of certain ocular diseases.

The immunologists, for their part, had their eyes literally opened by the realization that ocular diseases might be intrinsically interesting, and might offer useful models for the study of basic immunologic phenomena (one somnolent immunologist was observed to awaken wide-eyed during an ocular presentation to exclaim, "That's _very_ interesting."). In brief, the immunologist found himself fascinated by the problem of sympathetic ophthalmia, and the potential utility of the experimental model of auto-allergic disease that follows the injection of retinal antigens; he came to appreciate for the first time that the corneal graft may provide an almost unique system for the study of fundamental problems in transplant-ation biology; and he went away wondering why he had not heard earlier about such diseases as anterior uveitis and trachoma, and their implica-tions for the study of mechanisms of immunopathology and of antibody formation.

It is for all of these reasons and more that the participants of this symposium felt that it had been a thoroughly worthwhile and productive enterprise. It remains for me, on their behalf, to thank the Director and the staff of the National Eye Institute for having conceived of and supporting this type of conference. It is clear that those in attendance bene-

fitted greatly from the meeting. We may hope that the specific recommend-

ations to the Eye Institute that were developed at the conference will be

implemented, so as to extend these benefits even further within the field

of ophthalmic research.

DATE DUE			
GAYLORD			PRINTED IN U.S.A.